Visit our website

to find out about other books from Mosby
and our sister companies in Harcourt Health Sci

Register free at
www.harcourt-international.com

and you will get

- the latest information on new books, journals and electronic products in your chosen subject areas

- the choice of e-mail or post alerts or both, when there are any new books in your chosen areas

- news of special offers and promotions

- information about products from all Harcourt Health Sciences companies including Baillière Tindall, Churchill Livingstone, Mosby and W. B. Saunders

You will also find an easily searchable catalogue, online ordering, information on our extensive list of journals...and much more!

Visit the Harcourt Health Sciences website today!

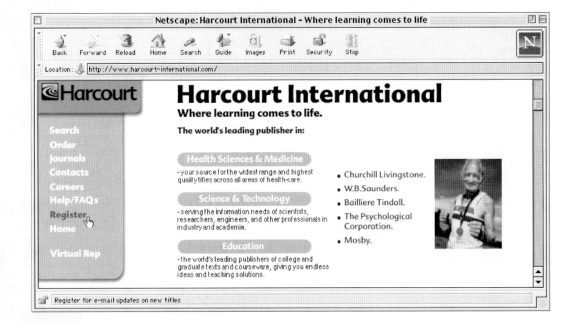

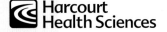

Color Atlas of

CLINICAL ANATOMY OF THE DOG & CAT

Commissioning Editor   Serena Bureau
Project Development Manager   Sheila Black
Project Manager   Rolla Couchman
Design Manager   Ian Dick
Production Manager   Helen Sofio

Color Atlas of

CLINICAL ANATOMY OF THE DOG & CAT

Second Edition

J S Boyd BVMS PhD MRCVS
Professor of Clinical Veterinary Anatomy
Department of Veterinary Preclinical Studies
Division of Veterinary Anatomy
The University of Glasgow Veterinary School
Bearsden, Glasgow

C Paterson MSc
Supervisor of Veterinary Ultrasound
Department of Veterinary Preclinical Studies
Division of Veterinary Anatomy
The University of Glasgow Veterinary School
Bearsden, Glasgow

with

A H May ARPS AMPA
Head Photographer
Faculty of Veterinary Medicine Information Service Unit
The University of Glasgow Veterinary School
Bearsden, Glasgow

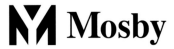

London • Edinburgh • New York • Philadelphia • St Louis • Sydney • Toronto 2001

MOSBY
An imprint of Mosby International Limited

© Mosby International Limited 2001

M is a registered trademark of Mosby International Limited

Second edition published 2001
First edition published 1991
Reprinted 1995
Reprinted 1999

ISBN 0 7234 3168 X

British Library Cataloguing in Publication Data
A catalogue record for this book is available from the British Library

Library of Congress Cataloging in Publication Data
A catalog record for this book is available from the Library of Congress

Note
Medical knowledge is constantly changing. As new information becomes available, changes in treatment, procedures, equipment and the use of drugs become necessary. The authors and the publishers have taken care to ensure that the information given in this text is accurate and up to date. However, readers are strongly advised to confirm that the information, especially with regard to drug usage, complies with the latest legislation and standards of practice.

Typeset by EXPO Holdings in Malaysia
Printed by Grafos SA, Arte sobre papel, Barcelona, Spain

The
Publisher's
policy is to use
**paper manufactured
from sustainable forests**

CONTENTS

ACKNOWLEDGEMENTS

The authors would most sincerely like to thank Allan May, whose great skill as a photographer made the production of this book possible. His endless patience and sense of humour brought pleasure to otherwise difficult and sometimes disappointing tasks.

The radiographs of the thorax, abdomen and spinal column were provided by radiographer Janice Lloyd, DCR, and a number of ultrasound and radiographic images were the work of Alison Dickie, BVMS, MVM, CVR, MRCVS. We are indebted to both of them for their contributions. The bone preparations were produced by Susan Cain, whom we thank for her skill and perseverance. The joint and distal limb dissections were the work of Fiona Patrick, BSc, whose dexterity was greatly appreciated.

We also wish to extend our gratitude to our respective wives, Isobel and Jean, for their forbearance and encouragement throughout the long hours of preparation of this book.

J S Boyd
C Paterson
2000

PREFACE

Instruction in veterinary anatomy is usually approached in one of two ways: in the initial stages of undergraduate teaching, the emphasis is mainly on structure and function, with a demand for greater detail of the individual organs, usually presented on a systems basis. At this stage, students use the standard texts that rely on illustrating the anatomical features by means of line diagrams. Later in their studies, the students become more aware of the importance of regional and topographical anatomy, where line diagrams may not fully illustrate the structures seen during dissection or clinical examination. For this reason, the greater topographical detail of a pictorial atlas is often preferred.

Veterinary anatomical atlases, past and present, have followed the conventions of human anatomical teaching, using either detailed artists' impressions or photographs of embalmed, dissected cadavers. The lack of realism, with the loss of normal colour and form, often detracts from these publications, as the specimens demonstrated so often bear little resemblance to the natural organs and tissues. Veterinary anatomy differs widely from its human counterpart in its ability to utilise fresh material. The veterinary clinician, surgeon or pathologist would much prefer to consult an anatomy atlas that presents with greater realism those structures encountered when examining or operating on a living animal, or when performing an autopsy. Greater demands are also being made of anatomical teaching to accommodate the newer imaging modalities, such as radiography and ultrasonography, where topographical and cross-sectional anatomy is becoming increasingly relevant.

This atlas provides photographic illustrations of the gross anatomy of the dog and cat, using, wherever possible, fresh, unprocessed material. Bony specimens have been presented in a more classical anatomical fashion, but they are displayed both singly and in articulated form, with areas of muscle attachment clearly outlined. The book begins with the head and works logically, on a regional basis, in a caudal direction. The osteology of each region is illustrated and the topography of the organs and structures is revealed, first in terms of living surface anatomy and then through a series of prepared dissections of fresh cadavers. The salient structures that appear in the photographs are numbered to correspond to the legends in order to assist identification, and also to facilitate self testing by the reader. Wherever pertinent, clinical and surgical features of note are also described alongside the photographs to enlarge upon the illustrated structures and regions. The degree of detail in the presentation of the vascular and neural supplies is deliberately restricted: only major vessels and nerve trunks are named when they are of particular interest in surgical fields or are of clinical importance. The radiographic features of each region are displayed and cross-sectional anatomical specimens are used, where appropriate, to demonstrate particular topographical planes. In certain regions, ultrasonographs of soft tissue structures are used for comparison with the cross-sectional anatomy.

Most of the photographs and the text refer to the anatomy of the dog, while cat anatomy is given a more comparative role, with morphological differences between the species being illustrated. The dissections have been prepared from fresh material, but all the cadavers used for the photographs were animals that had to undergo euthanasia for other reasons. No animal was sacrificed to provide illustrative material for this publication.

With the dissections, the policy has been to reveal structures in as natural a manner as possible: thus realism has been a greater consideration than stylised anatomical preparation. This type of approach has produced a veterinary anatomical atlas that shows that veterinary anatomy need no longer be limited to the examination of artificially prepared, embalmed specimens, but that it can serve the needs of those requiring realistic anatomical information when studying or practising veterinary medicine.

JS Boyd
C Peterson
2000

DEDICATION

To the memory of the late Helen J Smith,
MRCVS, former Head of the Department of
Veterinary Anatomy at Glasgow University
Veterinary School, who gave us our initial
and lasting enthusiasm for the study of
veterinary anatomy.

| INTRODUCTION

Without wishing to appear too pedantic, the consistent use of basic anatomical terminology is of paramount importance to permit proper communication not only among veterinary anatomists themselves, but also between anatomists and clinicians. To this end, a common nomenclature has been devised, *Nomina Anatomica Veterinaria* (NAV), that has greatly assisted in clarifying the channels of communication.

At first sight, the system may seem laboured, since the original NAV is in Latin, but it is quite permissible to use the same terms and names translated into English, as happens in many instances throughout the atlas. However, where muscles of the body appear in key lists, the Latin form has been retained to avoid a conflict in terminology. On a few occasions, an alternative term may appear after the standard NAV version, where an older name for a structure is still so widely used that it is regarded as common parlance.

When discussing topographical anatomy, the need for uniform description of both direction and position also becomes obvious. The photographs of the live dog in this chapter are annotated to demonstrate the standard directional and positional terms (**1–3**). Also included are a small number of regional names for specific areas of the body and limbs. Adjectives that have common usage in human anatomy, such as 'anterior', 'posterior', 'superior' and 'inferior', should not be employed in veterinary anatomy, except in a limited number of instances, to describe certain structures in the head region (e.g., within the eye or the brain).

In the live animal, standing erect on all four limbs, structures located towards the back (*dorsum*) of the animal are said to be 'dorsal' in position; this applies to the trunk, head and even the tail. The opposite of this position is termed 'ventral', describing structures that lie closest to the belly (*venter*) of the animal. Any structures that are located towards the head (*cranium*) are referred to as 'cranial', while those located towards the tail (*cauda*) are said to be 'caudal'. This system of identification requires finer definition in the head region itself, where the term 'rostral' is used for structures located closer to the muzzle (*rostrum*), rather than the broader term 'cranial'. However, the contrary direction in the head region is still termed 'caudal'.

The median (*medianus*) plane passes through the animal from head to tail, along the line of the vertebral column (*axis*), and divides the whole body into two symmetrical halves. Planes passing to either side of the median plane but parallel to it are referred to as 'sagittal'. However, sometimes, if the plane is close to the median, it is called 'paramedian'. The structures that lie closer to the median plane are said to be 'medial', while those that lie towards the outer side or flank (*latus*) of the animal are classified as 'lateral'. Sections of the head and trunk, that are parallel to the back (*dorsum*) of the animal are said to be in the dorsal plane, whereas sections made at right angles to the axis of the body are referred to as being 'transverse'.

The limbs require further definition and interpretation because their position may alter relative to the trunk. The proximal region of a limb is that closer to the trunk, while the area further from the trunk is distal. In the proximal region of the thoracic and pelvic limbs (i.e., down to the proximal limit of the carpus and tarsus) the area closer to the 'front' of the limb is cranial in contrast to the area closer to the 'rear', which is caudal. Distal to the carpus in the thoracic limb, the continuation of the cranial surface is termed 'dorsal' and that of the caudal surface is 'palmar'. With the pelvic limb, the equivalent terms for areas distal to the tarsus are 'dorsal' and 'plantar'. There is also a notional central axis running the length of each limb, and any section perpendicular to it is termed 'transverse'. If a structure in the limb lies closer to the central axis, it is 'axial' in position, in contrast to structures lying away from the central axis, which are 'abaxial'.

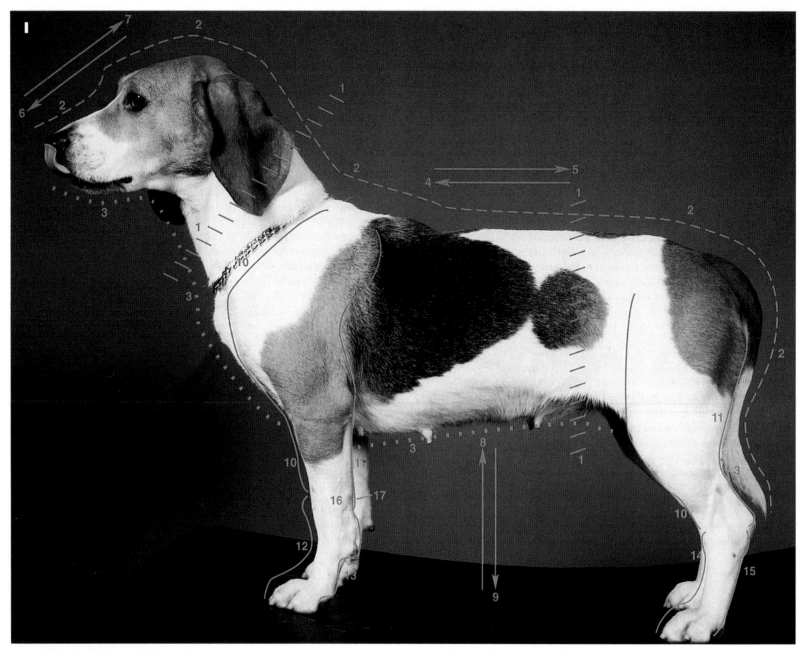

I   Lateral aspect of a standing live dog. The oblique dashes indicate the transverse plane, and the straight dashes, dots and continuous lines indicate the position and direction. Note, in particular, the specific terms for the head and the distal limbs.

1	Transverse plane of trunk	10	Cranial	proximal limb
2	Dorsal	11	Caudal	
3	Ventral	trunk and head	12	Dorsal	thoracic limb
4	Cranial	trunk	13	Palmar	(distal to carpus)
5	Caudal		14	Dorsal	pelvic limb
6	Rostral	head	15	Plantar	(distal to tarsus)
7	Caudal		16	Lateral	limb
8	Proximal	limb	17	Medial	
9	Distal				

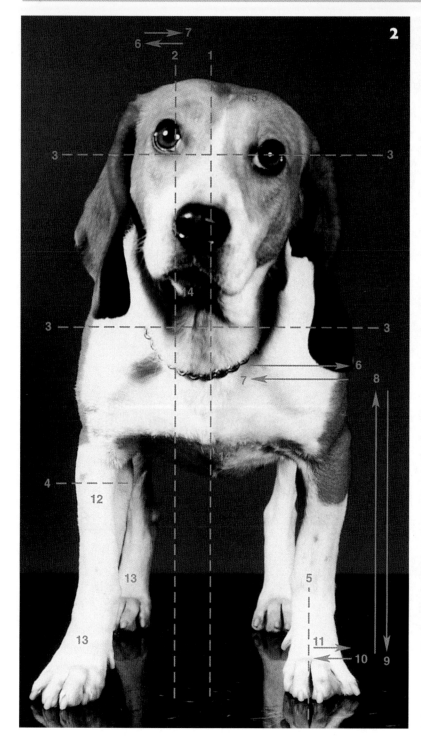

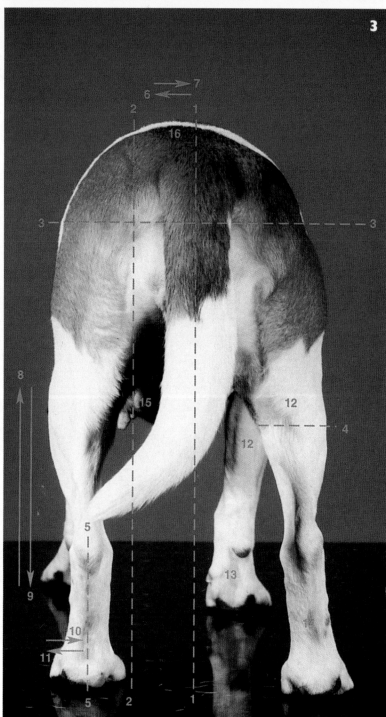

2   Cranial aspect of a standing live dog. The dotted lines indicate the anatomical planes of the body, and the arrows indicate the position and direction. Aspects of the head, trunk and limbs are marked by separate numbers.

3   Caudal aspect of a standing live dog. The dotted lines indicate the anatomical planes of the body, and the arrows indicate the position and direction. Aspects of the trunk and limbs are marked by separate numbers.

1	Median plane	8	Proximal	} limb
2	Sagittal plane	9	Distal	
3	Dorsal plane	10	Axial	
4	Transverse plane } of limb	11	Abaxial	
5	Axial plane	12	Cranial	} limb
6	Lateral	13	Dorsal	
7	Medial	14	Ventral	} trunk and head
		15	Dorsal	

1	Median plane	9	Distal	
2	Sagittal plane	10	Axial	
3	Dorsal plane	11	Abaxial	} limbs
4	Transverse plane } of limb	12	Caudal	
5	Axial plane	13	Palmar	
6	Lateral	14	Plantar	
7	Medial } limb	15	Ventral	} trunk
8	Proximal	16	Dorsal	

Clinical Note
Note that the term paramedian is sometimes applied to a sagittal plane that is close to the median plane.

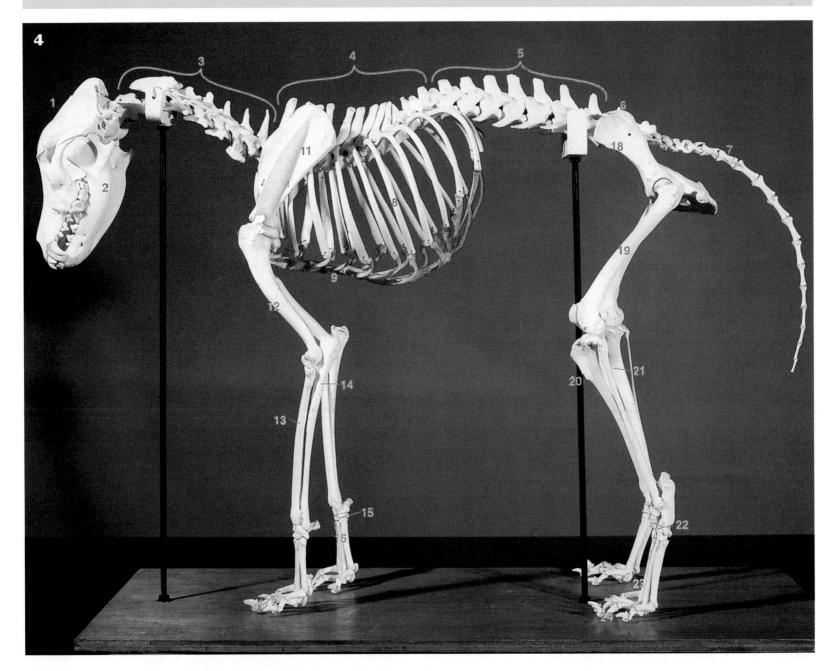

4   Lateral aspect of an articulated standing skeleton of a dog.

1	Skull	13	Radius
2	Mandible	14	Ulna
3	Cervical vertebrae	15	Carpus
4	Thoracic vertebrae	16	Metacarpus
5	Lumbar vertebrae	17	Phalanges
6	Sacrum	18	Ossa coxae
7	Caudal vertebrae	19	Femur
8	Ribs	20	Tibia
9	Sternum	21	Fibula
10	Costal arch	22	Tarsus
11	Scapula	23	Metatarsus
12	Humerus	24	Phalanges

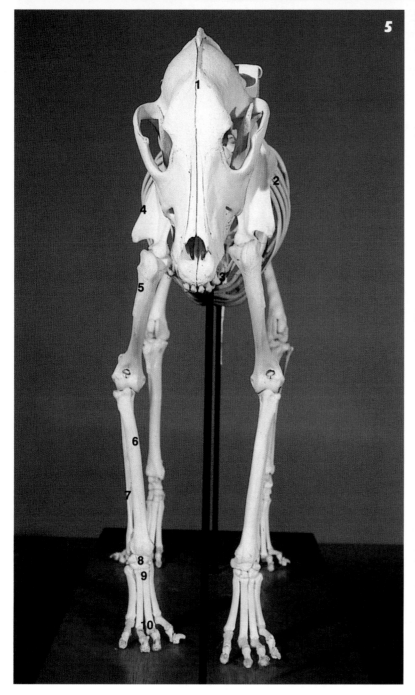

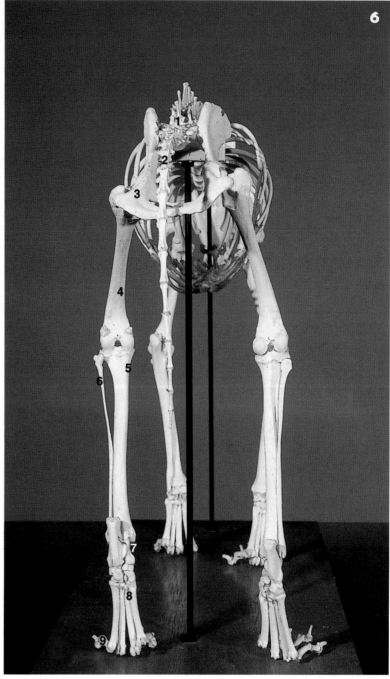

5   Cranial aspect of an articulated standing skeleton of a dog.

1	Skull	6	Radius
2	Ribs	7	Ulna
3	Sternum	8	Carpus
4	Scapula	9	Metacarpus
5	Humerus	10	Phalanges of manus

6   Caudal aspect of an articulated standing skeleton of a dog.

1	Sacrum	6	Fibula
2	Caudal vertebrae	7	Tarsus
3	Ossa coxae	8	Metatarsus
4	Femur	9	Phalanges of pes
5	Tibia		

2 HEAD AND NECK

Dealing with the structures of the head and neck, this chapter uses the live animal to indicate the palpable landmarks of the region, while the osteological features are demonstrated using bony specimens and radiographs.

Soft tissue structures are illustrated in detail, with a series of prepared dissections, and their topographical relationships are displayed by means of additional cross-sectional specimens and radiography.

7   Lateral aspect of the head and neck region of a live dog, demonstrating palpable landmarks.

1	Incisive bone	13	External sagittal crest
2	Infraorbital foramen	14	External occipital protuberance
3	Medial commissure of eyelids	15	Pinna of ear
4	Puncta lacrimale of upper lid (palpebra superior)	16	Zygomatic arch
5	Puncta lacrimale of lower lid (palpebra inferior)	17	M. masseter
6	Third eyelid	18	Angular process of mandible
7	Angular vein of the eye	19	Position of mandibular lymph nodes
8	Lateral commissure of eyelids	20	Body of mandible
9	Maxilla	21	Commissure of lips
10	Zygomatic process of frontal bone	22	Tongue (extruded)
11	M. temporalis	23	Larynx
12	Temporal line	24	External jugular (site for venepuncture)

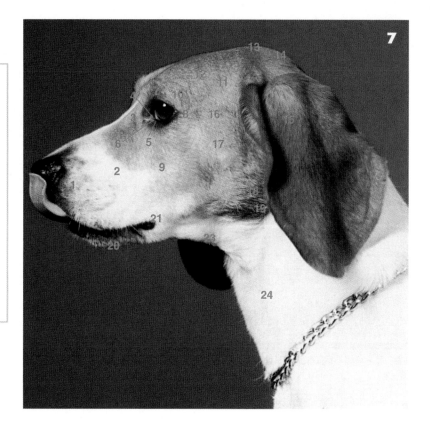

8   Cranial aspect of the head and neck region of a live dog, demonstrating palpable landmarks.

1	Planum nasale	11	Medial commissure of eyelids
2	Nares (nostril)	12	Third eyelid
3	Philtrum	13	Lateral commissure of eyelid
4	Upper lip (labia superior)	14	Zygomatic arch
5	Tactile hairs	15	Zygomatic process of frontal bone
6	Incisive bone	16	Frontal bone
7	Body of mandible	17	M. temporalis
8	Nasal bones	18	M. masseter
9	Maxilla	19	Pinna of ear
10	Infraorbital foramen		

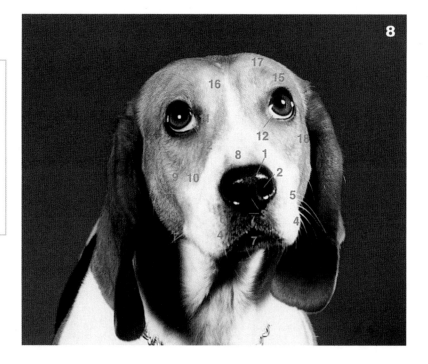

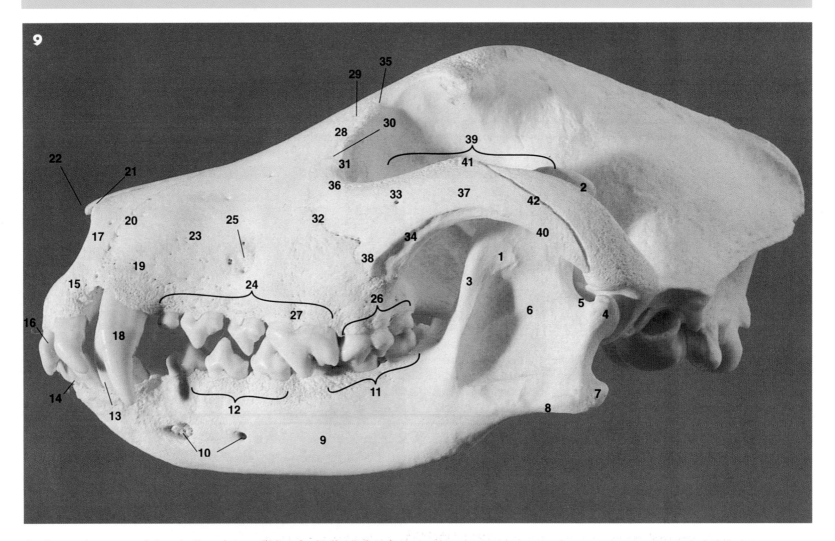

9   Lateral aspect of the skull and mandible of a bull terrier dog.

1	Ramus of mandible	15	Incisive bone	29	Frontomaxillary suture
2	Coronoid process	16	Upper incisor teeth	30	Lacrimomaxillary suture
3	Coronoid crest	17	Nasal process	31	Lacrimal bone
4	Condyloid process	18	Upper canine tooth	32	Zygomaticomaxillary suture
5	Mandibular notch	19	Alveolus of canine tooth	33	Infraorbital margin
6	Masseteric fossa	20	Incisivomaxillary suture	34	Masseteric margin
7	Angular process	21	Nasoincisive suture	35	Groove for angular vein of eye
8	Masseteric line	22	Nasal bone	36	Lacrimozygomatic suture
9	Body of mandible	23	Maxilla	37	Zygomatic bone
10	Mental foramina	24	Upper premolar teeth	38	Maxillary process
11	Lower molar teeth	25	Infraorbital foramen	39	Zygomatic arch
12	Lower premolar teeth	26	Upper molar teeth	40	Temporal process
13	Lower canine tooth	27	Alveolar juga	41	Frontal process
14	Lower incisor teeth	28	Frontal process	42	Temporozygomatic suture

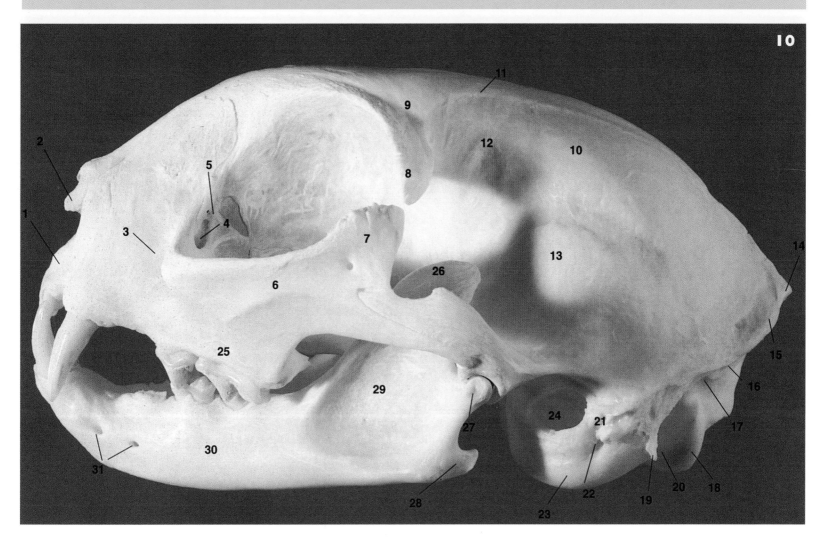

10   Lateral aspect of the skull and mandible of a cat.

1 Incisive bone	10 Parietal bone	21 Mastoid process
2 Nasal bone	11 Temporal line	22 Stylomastoid foramen
3 Infraorbital foramen	12 Temporal fossa	23 Tympanic bulla
4 Fossa for lacrimal sac	13 Squamous temporal bone	24 External acoustic meatus
5 Lacrimal bone	14 External occipital protuberance	25 Maxilla
6 Zygomatic bone	15 Nuchal crest	26 Coronoid process
7 Frontal process of zygomatic bone	16 Occipital bone	27 Condyloid process
8 Zygomatic process of frontal bone	17 Dorsal condyloid fossa	28 Angular process
	18 Occipital condyle	29 Masseteric fossa
9 Frontal bone	19 Jugular process	30 Body of mandible
	20 Ventral condyloid fossa	31 Mental foramina

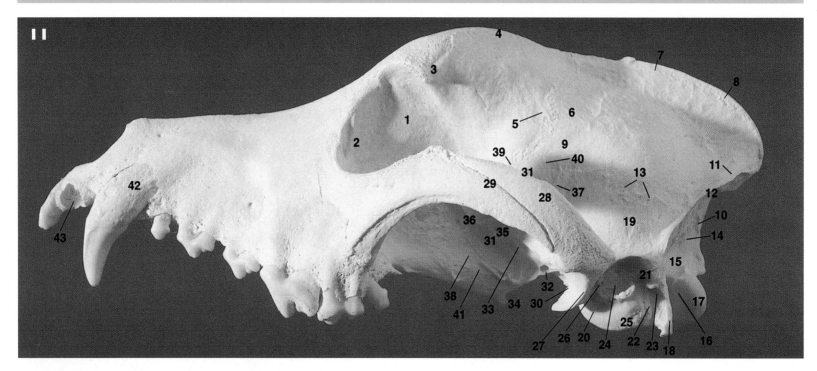

11

11   Lateral aspect of the skull of a dog, without the mandible.

1 Frontal bone	11 Occipitoparietal suture	23 Stylomastoid foramen	35 Orbital fissure
2 Fossa for lacrimal gland	12 Nuchal line	24 External acoustic meatus	36 Orbital canal
3 Zygomatic process of 1	13 Squamous suture	25 Tympanic bulla	37 Sphenosquamous suture
4 Temporal line	14 Mastoid foremen	26 Retroarticular foramen	38 Sphenopalatine suture
5 Frontoparietal suture (coronal	15 Dorsal condyloid fossa	27 Retroarticular process	39 Sphenofrontal suture
suture)	16 Ventral condyloid fossa	28 Zygomatic process	40 Sphenoparietal suture
6 Parietal bone	17 Occipital condyle	29 Temporozygomatic suture	41 Pterygosphenoid suture
7 External sagittal crest	18 Jugular process	30 Mandibular fossa	42 Alveolus of canine tooth
8 Interparietal process and	19 Squamous ⎫ part of temporal	31 Sphenoid bone	(lateral wall partially resected)
parietointerparietal suture	20 Tympanic ⎭ bone	32 Caudal alar foramen	43 Alveolus of incisor tooth
9 Temporal fossa	21 Mastoid process	33 Rostral alar foramen	
10 Occipital bone	22 Tympano-occipital suture	34 Pterygoid bone	

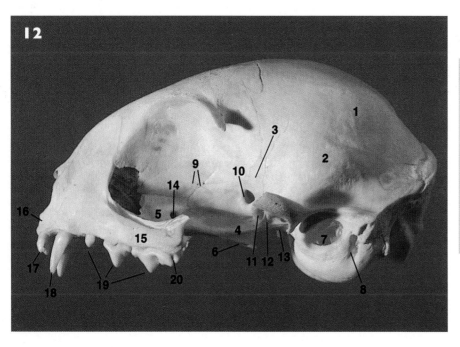

12

12   Lateral aspect of the skull of a cat. The zygomatic arch has been removed from the left side.

1 Parietal bone	10 Optic canal
2 Squamous temporal	11 Orbital fissure
bone	12 Rostral alar foramen
3 Wing of basisphenoid	13 Caudal alar foramen
bone	14 Sphenopalatine foramen
4 Presphenoid bone	15 Maxilla
5 Palatine bone	16 Incisive bone
6 Pterygoid bone	17 Incisor teeth
7 External acoustic meatus	18 Canine tooth
8 Stylomastoid foramen	19 Premolar teeth
9 Ethmoid foramina	20 Molar tooth

13 Medial aspect of a sagittal section of the left half of the skull of a cat.

1 Parietal bone
2 Frontal bone
3 Frontal sinus
4 Ethmoturbinates
5 Cribriform plate
6 Ethmoidal foramina
7 Nasal bone
8 Dorsal nasal concha
9 Ventral nasal concha
10 Incisive bone
11 Maxilla
12 Vomer
13 Alveoli of third premolar and first molar
14 Sphenoidal sinus
15 Presphenoid bone
16 Basisphenoid bone
17 Optic canal
18 Dorsum sellae
19 Tentorium osseum
20 Internal acoustic meatus
21 Jugular foramen
22 Hypoglossal canal
23 Occipital bone

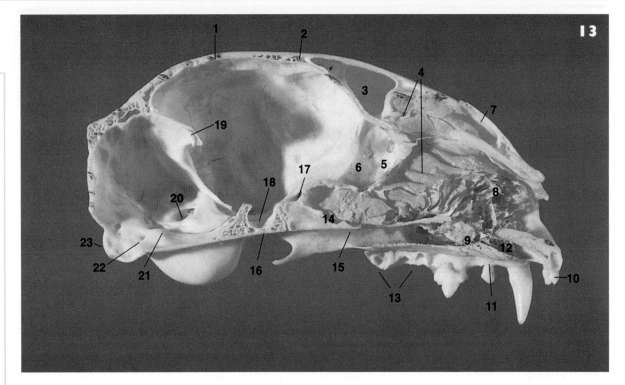

14 Dorsal aspect of the skull of a cat.

1 Incisive bone
2 Nasal bone
3 Maxilla
4 Frontal bone
5 Zygomatic process of frontal bone
6 Zygomatic bone
7 Frontal process

8 Coronoid process of mandible
9 Temporal bone
10 Zygomatic process of temporal bone
11 Parietal bone
12 Interparietal bone
13 Sagittal crest
14 Occipital bone

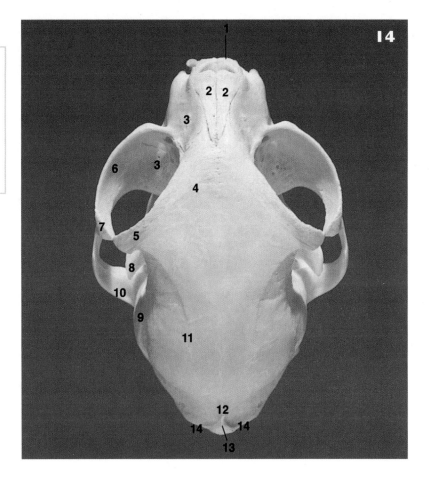

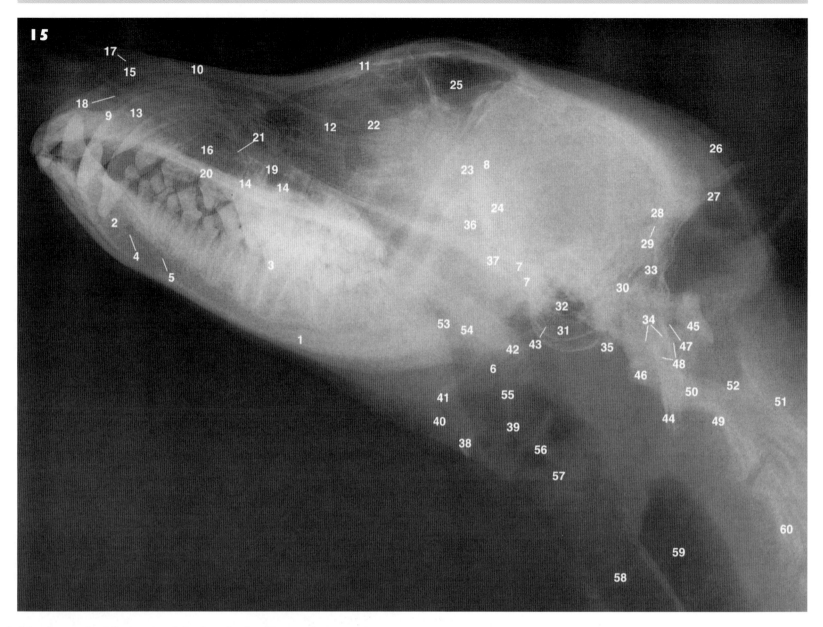

15   Lateral radiograph of the head of a dog.

1 Mandible	17 Dorsal nasal meatus	31 Tympanic bulla	46 Ventral arch
2 Lower canine	18 Ventral nasal meatus	32 External acoustic meatus	47 Intervertebral foramen
3 First lower molar	19 Maxillary sinus	33 Condyloid fossa	48 Transverse foramen
4 Mental foramina	20 Hard palate	34 Occipital condyle	49 Body {of second cervical
5 Mandibular canal	21 Infraorbital foramen	35 Jugular process	vertebra (axis)
6 Angular process	22 Orbit	36 Presphenoid bone	50 Dens (odontoid process)
7 Condyloid process	23 Temporal process of zygomatic	37 Pterygoid process	51 Spinous process
8 Coronoid process	bone	38 Basihyoid bone	52 Cranial vertebral notch
9 Incisive bone	24 Zygomatic process of	39 Thyrohyoid bone	53 Root of tongue
10 Nasal bone	temporal bone	40 Keratohyoid bone	54 Soft palate
11 Frontal bone	25 Frontal sinus	41 Epihyoid bone	55 Epiglottis
12 Maxilla	26 Sagittal crest	42 Stylohyoid bone	56 Thyroid cartilage
13 Upper canine	27 External occipital protuberance	43 Tympanohyoid cartilage	57 Cricoid cartilage
14 Fourth upper premolar	28 Tentorium cerebelli osseum	44 Transverse process of first	58 Trachea
15 Dorsal nasal concha	29 Transverse canal	cervical vertebra (atlas)	59 Oesophagus
16 Ventral nasal concha	30 Petrous temporal bone	45 Dorsal arch	60 Third cervical vertebra

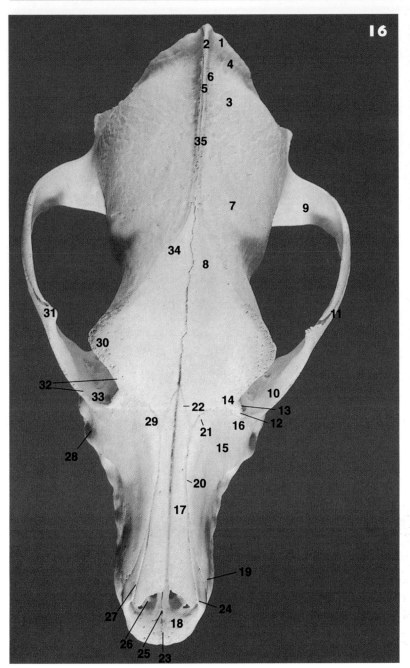

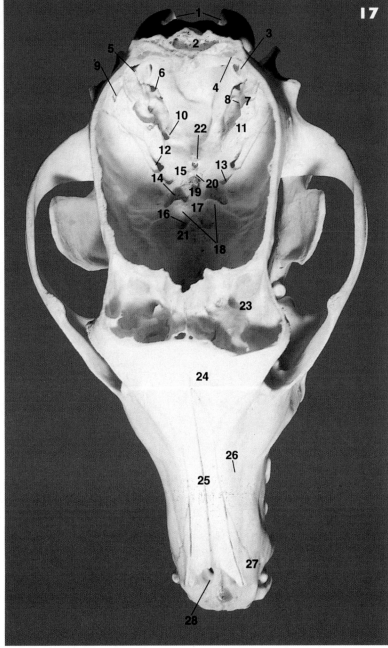

16   Dorsal aspect of the skull of a dog.

17   Dorsal aspect of the skull of a dog, with the dorsal calvaria removed. The angulation reveals the caudal structures of the cranial vault.

1 Occiptal bone	18 Incisive bone
2 Interparietal bone	19 Incisivomaxillary suture
3 Parietal bone	20 Nasomaxillary suture
4 Occipitoparietal suture	21 Frontomaxillary suture
5 Sagittal suture	22 Frontonasal suture
6 Parietointerparietal suture	23 Interincisive suture
7 Parietofrontal or coronal suture	24 Nasoincisive suture
8 Frontal bone	25 Incisive canal
9 Squamous part of temporal bone	26 Palatine fissure
10 Zygomatic bone	27 Nasal process of 18
11 Temporozygomatic bone	28 Infraorbital foramen
12 Lacrimal bone	29 Frontal process of 15
13 Lacrimozygomatic suture	30 Zygomatic process of 8 (supraorbital process)
14 Frontolacrimal suture	31 Frontal process of 10
15 Maxilla	32 Orbital margin
16 Lacrimomaxillary suture	33 Fossa for lacrimal sac
17 Nasal bone	34 Temporal line
	35 External sagittal crest

1 Occipital bone	15 Presphenoid bone
2 Transverse canal	16 Optic canal
3 Condyloid canal	17 Sulcus chiasmatis
4 Hypoglossal canal	18 Rostral clinoid process
5 Mastoid foramen	19 Hypophyseal fossa
6 Jugular foramen	20 Caudal clinoid process
7 Cerebellar fossa	21 Basisphenoid bone
8 Internal acoustic meatus	22 Dorsum sellae
9 Canal for transverse sinus	23 Frontal sinus (lateral part)
10 Canal for trigeminal nerve	24 Frontal bone
11 Crista partis petrosae	25 Nasal bone
12 Foramen ovale	26 Maxilla
13 Foramen rotundum	27 Incisive bone
14 Orbital fissure	28 Palatine fissure

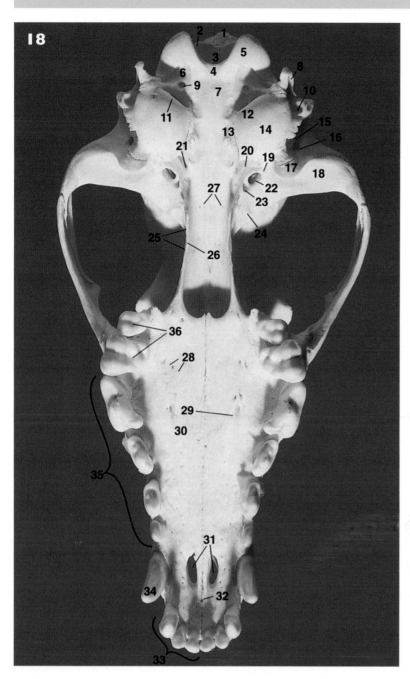

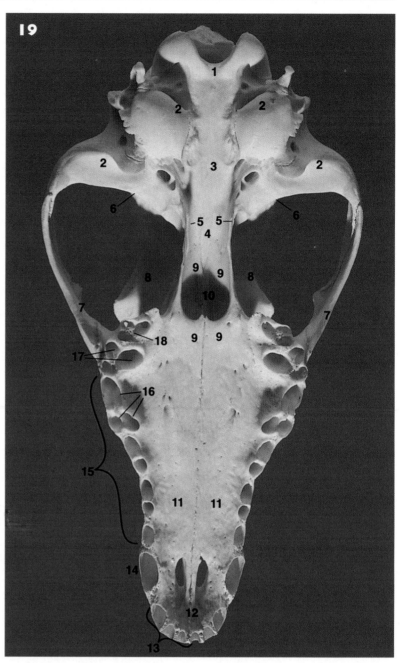

18   Ventral aspect of the skull of a dog, showing the upper dental arches.

19   Ventral aspect of the skull of a dog. The upper teeth have been removed to reveal the alveolar pattern of the upper dental arch.

1	External occipital protuberance	20	Foramen lacerum
2	Nuchal tubercle	21	Musculotubal canal
3	Foramen magnum	22	Foramen ovale with spinous
4	Intercondyloid incisure		foramen
5	Condyloid process	23	Caudal alar foramen
6	Ventral condyloid fossa	24	Rostral alar foramen
7	Pharyngeal tubercle	25	Orbital fissure
8	Jugular process	26	Optic canal
9	Hypoglossal canal	27	Caudal foramen of pterygoid
10	Stylomastoid foramen		canal
11	Tympano-occipital fissure	28	Minor palatine foramen
12	Jugular foramen	29	Major palatine foramen
13	Muscular tubercle	30	Palatine sulcus
14	Tympanic bulla	31	Palatine fissure
15	External acoustic meatus	32	Incisive canal
16	Temporal meatus	33	Incisor teeth
17	Retroarticular process	34	Canine tooth
18	Mandibular fossa	35	Premolar teeth
19	Petrotympanic fissure	36	Molar teeth

1	Occipital bone	11	Maxilla
2	Temporal bone	12	Incisive bone
3	Basisphenoid bone	13	Alveoli of incisor teeth
4	Presphenoid bone	14	Alveolus of canine tooth
5	Pterygoid bone	15	Alveoli of premolar teeth
6	Parietal bone	16	Alveolus of fourth premolar
7	Zygomatic bone		tooth
8	Frontal bone	17	Alveolus of first molar tooth
9	Palatine bone	18	Alveolus of second molar
10	Vomer		tooth

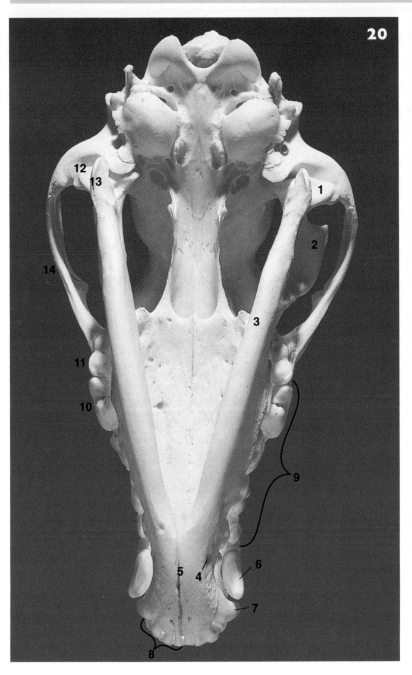

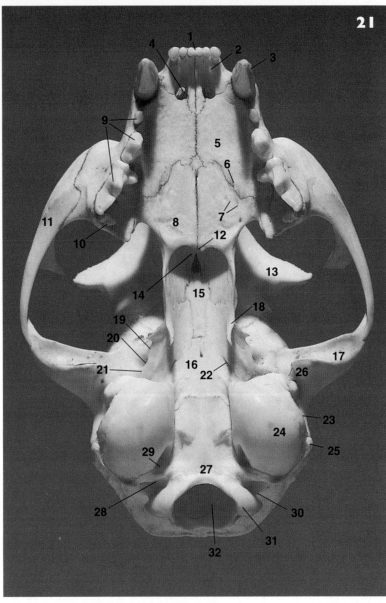

20   Ventral aspect of the skull and mandible of a dog.

1 Condyloid process	8 Lower incisor tooth
2 Coronoid process	9 Upper premolar teeth
3 Body of mandible	10 Fourth upper premolar tooth
4 Mental foramina	11 First upper molar tooth
5 Mandibular symphysis	12 Temporomandibular joint
6 Upper canine tooth	13 Angular process
7 Lower canine tooth	14 Zygomatic arch

21   Ventral aspect of the skull of a cat. A marker dye has been used to highlight the suture lines.

1 Incisor teeth	18 Hamulus of pterygoid
2 Incisive bone	19 Rostral alar foramen
3 Canine tooth	20 Caudal alar foramen
4 Palatine fissure	21 Foramen ovale
5 Maxilla	22 Pterygoid canal
6 Major palatine foramen	23 External acoustic meatus
7 Minor palatine foramina	24 Tympanic bulla
8 Palatine bone	25 Stylomastoid foramen
9 Premolar teeth	26 Retroarticular process
10 Molar tooth	27 Occipital bone
11 Zygomatic bone	28 Jugular process
12 Caudal nasal spine of 8	29 Jugular foramen
13 Frontal bone	30 Ventral condyloid fossa
14 Vomer	31 Occipital condyle (condyloid
15 Presphenoid bone	process)
16 Basisphenoid bone	32 Foramen magnum
17 Mandibular fossa	

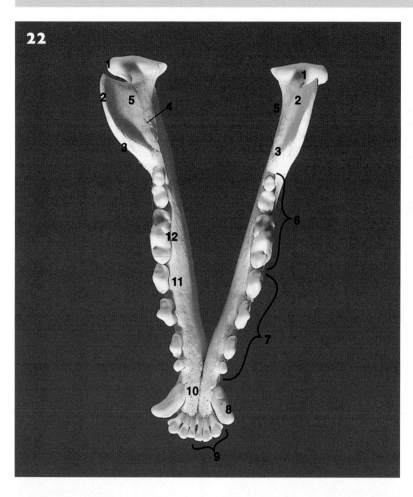

22   Dorsal aspect of the mandible of a dog.

   1 Condyloid process
   2 Coronoid process
   3 Coronoid crest
   4 Mandibular foramen
   5 Ramus of mandible
   6 Lower molar teeth
   7 Lower premolar teeth
   8 Lower canine tooth
   9 Lower incisor teeth
  10 Mandibular symphysis
  11 Body of mandible
  12 Mylohyoid crest

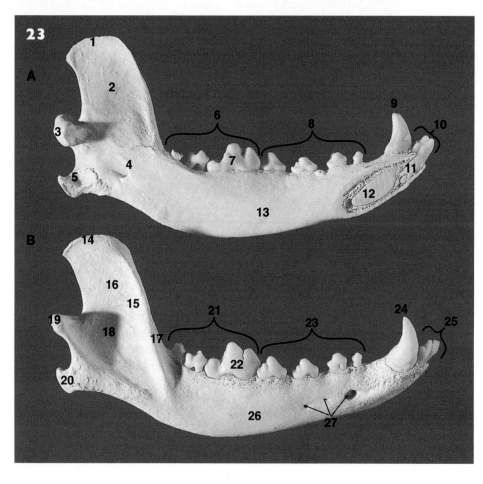

23   Medial (A) and lateral (B) aspect of the mandible of a dog.

   1 Coronoid process
   2 Ramus of mandible
   3 Condyloid process
   4 Mandibular foramen
   5 Angular process
   6 Molar teeth
   7 First molar tooth
   8 Premolar teeth
   9 Canine tooth
  10 Incisor teeth
  11 Alveolus of incisor tooth
  12 Canine root in alveolus
  13 Body of mandible
  14 Coronoid process
  15 Coronoid crest
  16 Ramus
  17 Mandibular notch
  18 Masseteric fossa
  19 Condyloid process
  20 Angular process
  21 Molar teeth
  22 First molar tooth
  23 Premolar teeth
  24 Canine tooth
  25 Incisor teeth
  26 Body of mandible
  27 Mental foramina

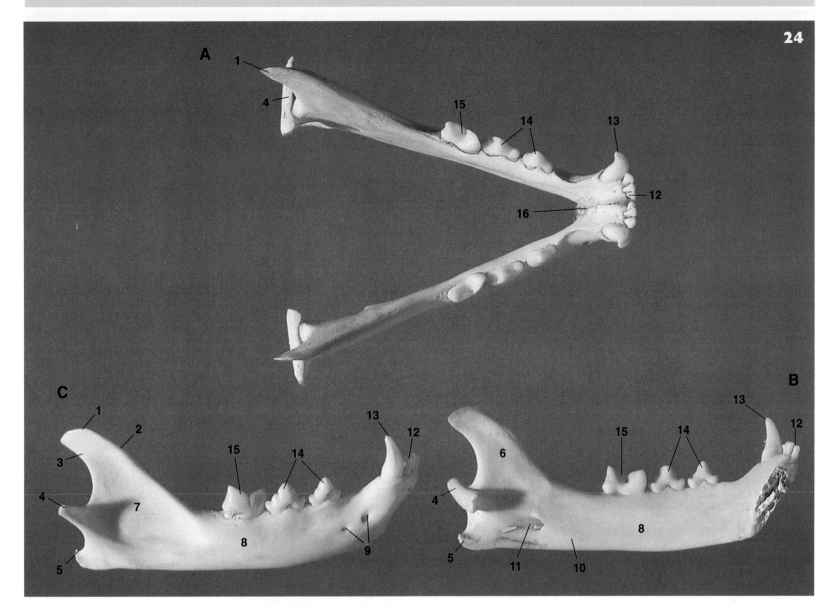

24   Dorsal aspect (A) of the left and right mandibles, medial aspect (B) of the left mandible and lateral aspect (C) of the right mandible of a cat.

1 Coronoid process	9 Mental foramina
2 Coronoid crest	10 Mylohyoid crest
3 Mandibular notch	11 Mandibular foramen
4 Condyloid process	12 Incisor teeth
5 Angular process	13 Canine tooth
6 Ramus of mandible	14 Premolar teeth
7 Masseteric fossa	15 Molar tooth
8 Body of mandible	16 Mandibular symphysis

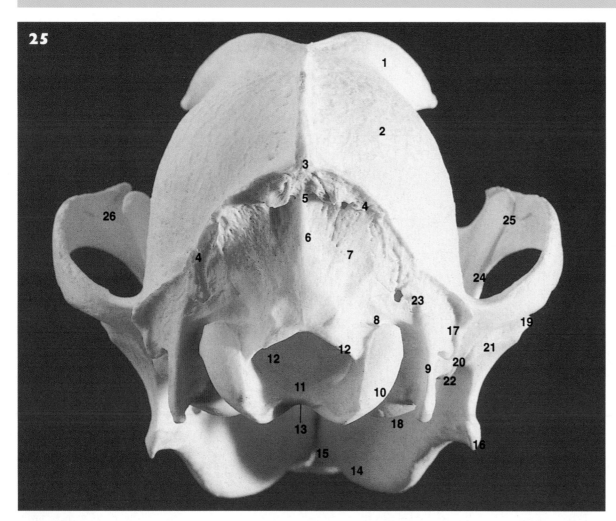

25   Caudal aspect of the skull and mandible of a dog.

1	Frontal bone
2	Parietal bone
3	Interparietal bone
4	Nuchal crest
5	External occipital protuberance
6	External occipital crest
7	Supraoccipital bone
8	Exoccipital bone
9	Jugular process
10	Occipital condyle
11	Foramen magnum
12	Nuchal tubercle
13	Intercondyloid notch
14	Body of mandible
15	Mandibular symphysis
16	Angular process
17	Temporal bone
18	Tympanic bulla
19	Zygomatic process
20	Mastoid process
21	Temporomandibular joint
22	Area of attachment of tympanohyoid
23	Mastoid foramen
24	Ramus of mandible
25	Coronoid process
26	Zygomatic bone

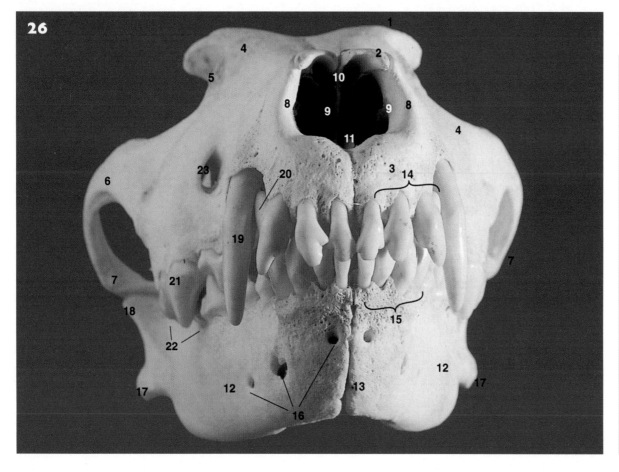

26   Rostral aspect of the skull and mandible of a dog.

1	Frontal bone
2	Nasal bone
3	Incisive bone
4	Maxilla
5	Lacrimal bone
6	Zygomatic bone
7	Zygomatic process of temporal bone
8	Osseous nasal opening
9	Nasal fossae
10	Nasal septum
11	Vomer
12	Body of mandible
13	Mandibular symphysis
14	Upper incisor teeth
15	Lower incisor teeth
16	Mental foramina
17	Angular process
18	Temporomandibular joint
19	Upper canine tooth
20	Lower canine tooth
21	Fourth upper premolar tooth
22	First lower molar tooth
23	Infraorbital foramen

27   Frontomandibular radiograph of the head of a dog.

1   Spinous process of second cervical vertebra (axis)
2   Dens (odontoid process)
3   Cranial articular surface
4   Transverse process of first cervical vertebral (atlas)
5   Alar notch
6   Transverse foramen
7   Caudal articular surface
8   Cranial articular surface
9   Nuchal line
10   Nuchal tubercle
11   Occipital condyle
12   Foramen magnum
13   Jugular process
14   Mastoid process
15   Petrous temporal bone
16   Crista partis petrosae
17   Tympanic bulla
18   External acoustic meatus
19   Hypophyseal fossa
20   Optic canal
21   Ethmoid fossa
22   Pterygoid process
23   Ethmoturbinates
24   Frontal sinus
25   Vomer
26   Palatine fissure
27   Medial wall of orbit
28   Zygomatic arch
29   Frontal process of zygomatic bone
30   Condyloid process
31   Angular process
32   Body of mandible
33   Coronoid process
34   Fourth upper premolar tooth
35   Upper canine tooth
36   Lower canine tooth

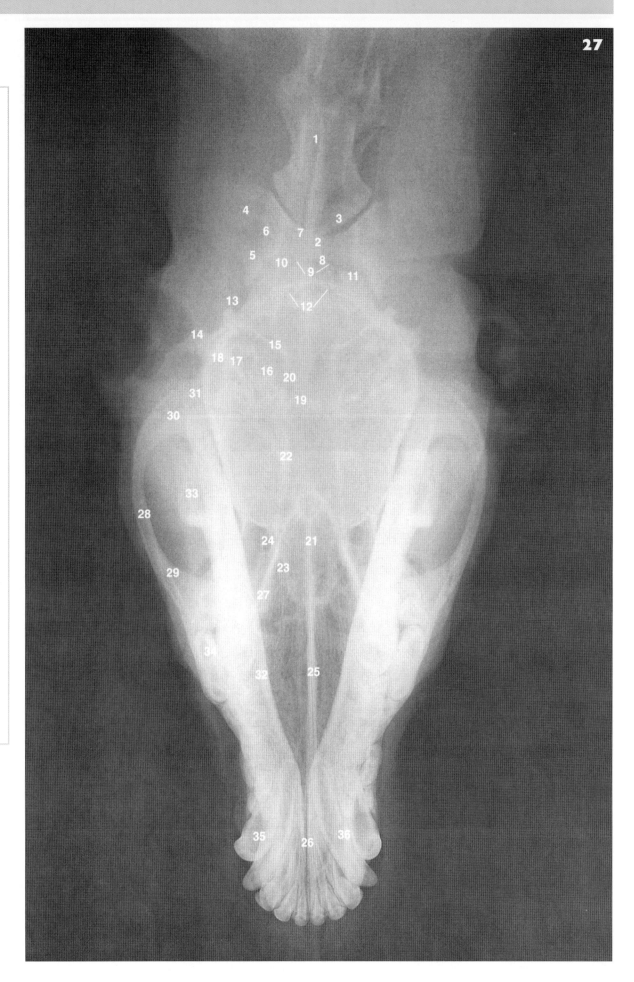

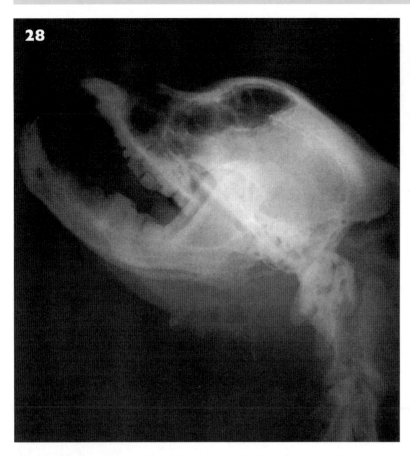

28 Lateral radiograph of the head of a brachycephalic breed of dog, demonstrating the greatly foreshortened facial portion of the skull.

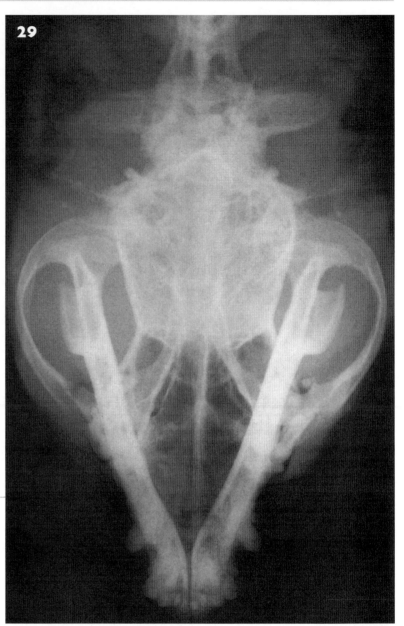

29 Mandibulofrontal radiograph of the head of brachycephalic breed of dog, demonstrating the malocclusion of the upper and lower dental arches.

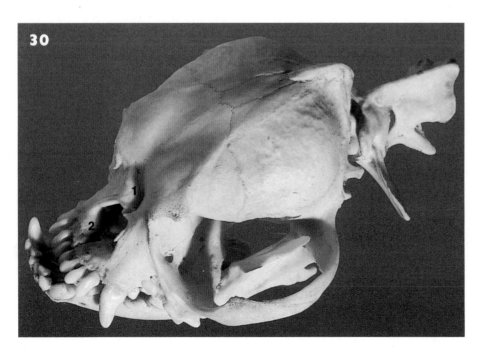

30 Dorsolateral aspect of the skull of a brachycephalic breed of dog, demonstrating the foreshortened facial region and the malocclusion of the dental arcade.

1	Frontal fossa
2	External nasal opening

31 Lateral aspect of a dolichocephalic skull of a dog, demonstrating the elongation of the facial region. There is an increased space between the canine and first premolar tooth (diastema).

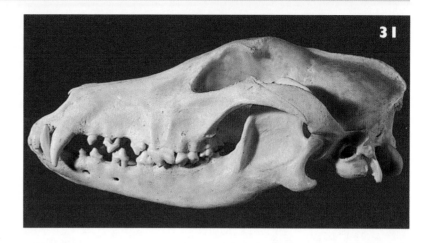

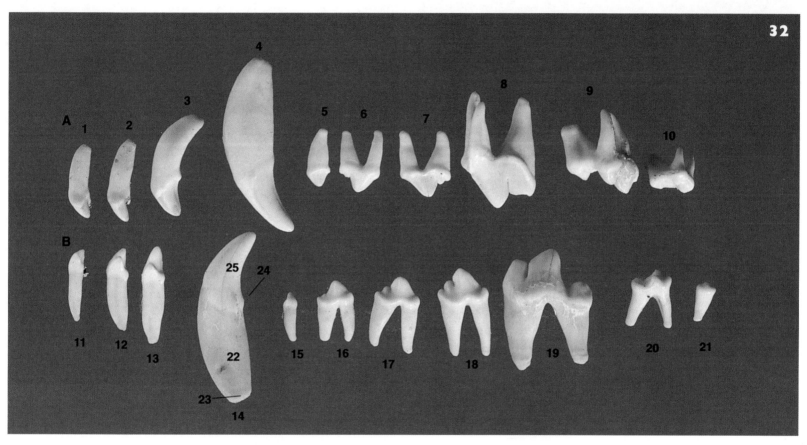

32 Dental arcade of an adult dog, showing the individual teeth from the upper (A) and lower (B) dental arch of the left half of a dog skull and mandible. Permanent dentition: $2\{I\frac{3}{3}\, C\frac{1}{1}\, P\frac{4}{4}\, M\frac{2}{3}\} = 42$. Deciduous dentition: $2\{Di\frac{3}{3}\, Dc\frac{1}{1}\, Dp\frac{3}{3}\} = 28$.

1	First	upper incisor tooth	
2	Second		
3	Third		
4	Upper canine tooth		
5	First	upper premolar tooth	
6	Second		
7	Third		
8	Fourth (carnassial)		
9	First	upper molar tooth	
10	Second		
11	First	lower incisor tooth	
12	Second		
13	Third		

14	Lower canine tooth		
15	First	lower premolar tooth	
16	Second		
17	Third		
18	Fourth		
19	First	lower molar tooth	
20	Second		
21	Third		
22	Root covered in cementum		
23	Apex of root		
24	Neck		
25	Crown covered in enamel		

Clinical Note

4 Note the wide diameter of the root of the adult canine tooth. This diameter is greater than the periphery of the alveolus at the gum margin, making it dangerous to apply direct traction to remove the tooth. The alveolar margin may be enlarged using a dental elevator or the lateral wall of the alveolus may be broken down, permitting the tooth to be lifted from the alveolus.

8 & 19 The upper 4th premolar and lower 1st molar teeth are the carnassial or sectorial teeth. The food is moved to the cheek region and is suspended between these teeth, which have a scissor-like effect, facilitating the severing of larger portions of meat. The upper carnassial (**8**) has a trifid root system which presents problems in extraction. The widespread nature of the root system necessitates the use of a dental elevator to loosen the tooth within the alveolus before extraction is possible.

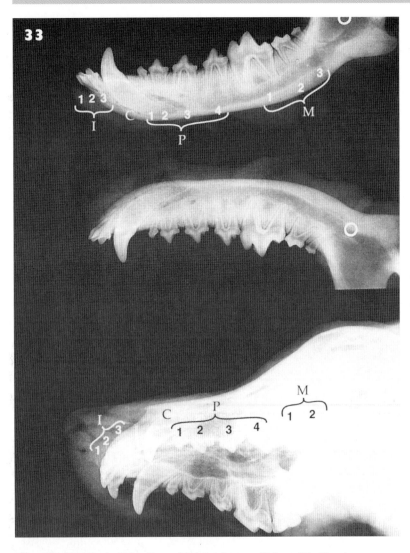

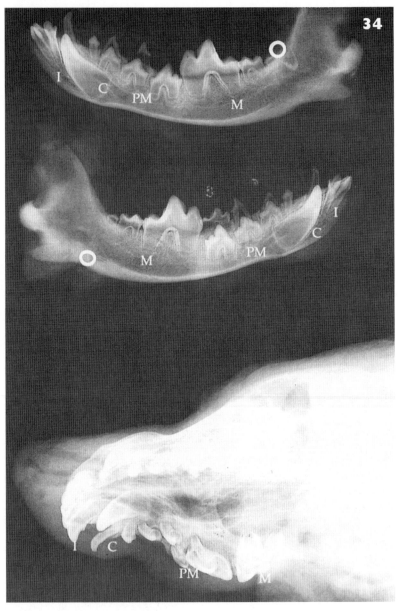

33   Radiograph of a disarticulated mandible with the two bodies separated, and an obliquely positioned skull, demonstrating the root formation of the adult canine dentition.

C	Canine tooth
I	Incisor teeth
P/PM	Premolar teeth
M	Molar teeth

34   Radiograph of the disarticulated and divided mandible and the obliquely positioned skull of a puppy, demonstrating the replacement of the deciduous dentition by the permanent dental arches. The deciduous incisors have been lost and the deciduous canines and premolars can be seen above their permanent replacements. Note that the first premolar occurs in the deciduous arch, but remains as a permanent tooth.

35 **Dental arcade of an adult cat, showing the individual teeth from the upper (A) and lower (B) dental arch.**

1 Incisor teeth
2 Canine tooth
3 Premolar teeth
4 Molar tooth

Clinical Note
Permanent dentition:
$$2 \left\{ I\, \tfrac{3}{3}\ C\, \tfrac{1}{1}\ P\, \tfrac{3}{2}\ M\, \tfrac{1}{1} \right\} = 30$$
The third upper premolar and first lower molar are the sectorial teeth.

Deciduous dentition:
$$2 \left\{ Di\, \tfrac{3}{3}\ Dc\, \tfrac{1}{1}\ Dp\, \tfrac{3}{2} \right\} = 26$$

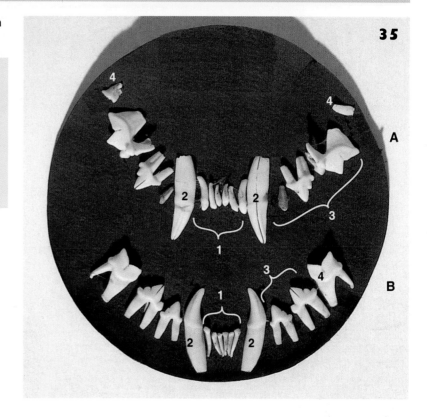

36 **Lateral aspect of the head of a dog. Only the skin has been resected to reveal the superficial muscles.**

1 M. platysma
2 M. sphincter colli superficialis
3 External jugular vein
4 M. parotidoauricularis
5 M. zygomaticoauricularis
6 Mm. cervicoauricularis
7 M. sphincter colli profundus
8 M. zygomaticus
9 M. orbicularis oris
10 M. levator nasolabialis
11 M. frontalis
12 M. orbicularis oculi
13 M. retractor anguli oculi lateralis
14 M. scutuloauricularis
15 Palpebral nerve (VII)
16 Zygomaticotemporal nerve (V)

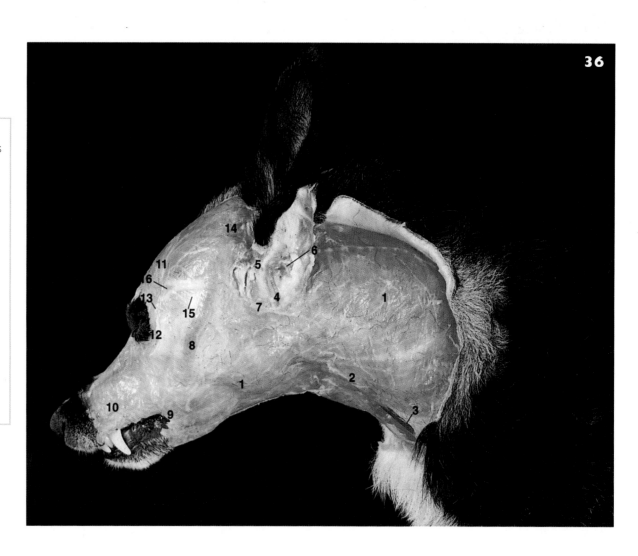

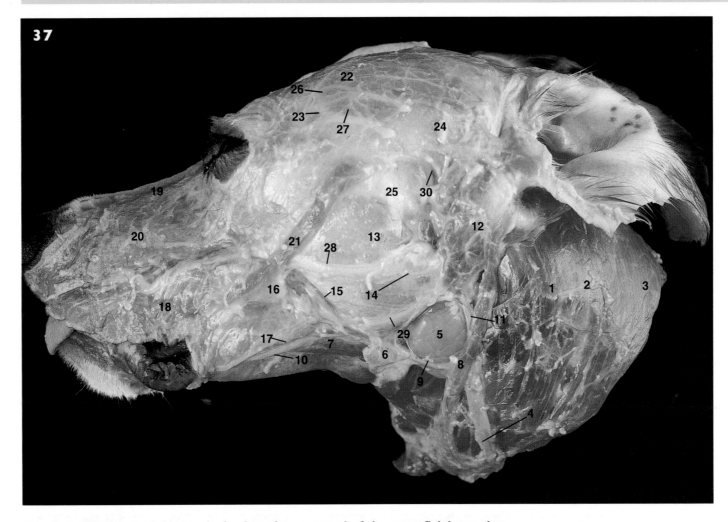

37

37   Lateral aspect of the head of a dog after removal of the superficial muscles.

1	M. sternomastoideus	16	M. buccinator
2	M. sterno-occipitalis	17	Lingual vein
3	M. cleidocervicalis	18	M. orbicularis oris
4	External jugular vein	19	M. levator nasolabialis
5	Mandibular salivary gland	20	M. levator labii maxillaris
6	Mandibular lymph node	21	M. zygomaticus
7	M. digastricus	22	M. frontalis
8	M. parotidoauricularis	23	M. retractor anguli oculi lateralis
9	Linguofacial vein	24	M. temporalis
10	M. mylohyoideus	25	Zygomatic arch
11	Maxillary vein	26	Zygomaticotemporal nerve (V)
12	Parotid salivary gland	27	Palpebral nerve (VII)
13	M. masseter	28	Dorsal buccal branch (VII)
14	Parotid duct	29	Ventral buccal branch (VII)
15	Facial vein	30	Auriculotemporal nerve (V)

Clinical Note

5   This is labelled as the mandibular salivary gland but in reality the structure incorporates both the mandibular gland and the monostomatic portion of the sublingual salivary gland. The two glands have separate ducts which run alongside each other deep to the M. digastricus and the body of the mandible.

6   This lymph node is normally palpable in the live dog and is used routinely in clinical examinations. Note its relationship to the division of the linguofacial vein and do not confuse it with the larger mandibular salivary gland which lies more dorsal in position.

12   Note the position of this gland relative to the cartilaginous external ear canal. During surgery to resect the vertical portion of the ear canal the parotid salivary gland is vulnerable to damage due to its proximity to the canal.

14   Note the position and course of the parotid duct. By resecting its oral opening into the buccal cavity at the level of the 4th upper premolar tooth this duct can be transplanted from its situation on the lateral facial region to be inserted into the upper lateral angle of the eye in an attempt to overcome the lack of tear secretion in the condition keratoconjunctivitis sicca (KCS).

38   Dorsal aspect of the superficial muscles of the head of a dog.

1 M. cervicoscutularis	9 M. retractor anguli oculi lateralis
2 M. cervicoauricularis	10 M. levator anguli oculi medialis
3 Cutaneous branch of second cervical nerve	11 M. levator nasolabialis
	12 Planum nasale
4 M. interscutularis	13 Palpebral rim
5 M. frontalis (cut edge)	14 Palpebral nerve (VII)
6 M. scutuloauricularis (cut edge)	15 Branches of rostral auricular nerve (VII)
7 M. zygomaticus	
8 M. orbicularis occuli	16 M. temporalis

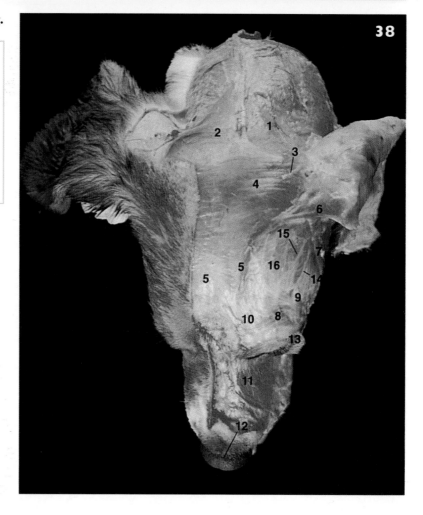

39   Lateral aspect of the muscles of the head of a dog after removal of the skin and cutaneous muscles.

1 M. temporalis
2 Superficial ⎤ part of
3 Middle ⎦ M. masseter
4 M. digastricus
5 M. stylohyoideus
6 Retropharyngeal lymph node
7 M. thyropharyngeus
8 M. thyrohyoideus
9 M. sternohyoideus
10 M. sternothyroideus
11 M. sternomastoideus ⎤ M. sterno-
12 M. sterno-occipitalis ⎦ cephalicus
13 M. cleidocervicalis
14 M. mylohyoideus
15 M. buccinator
16 M. retractor anguli oculi lateralis
17 M. frontalis (cut edge)

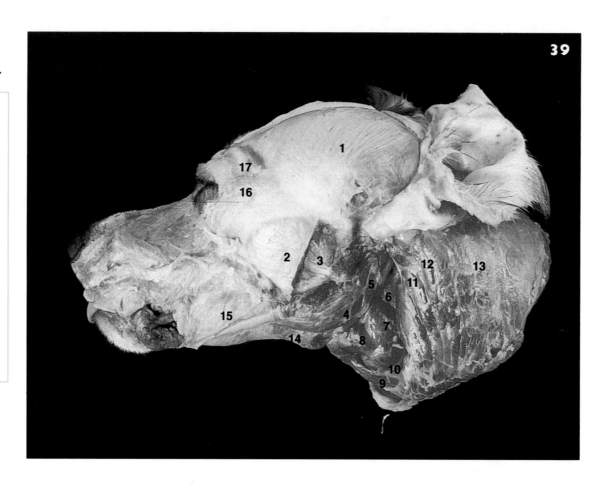

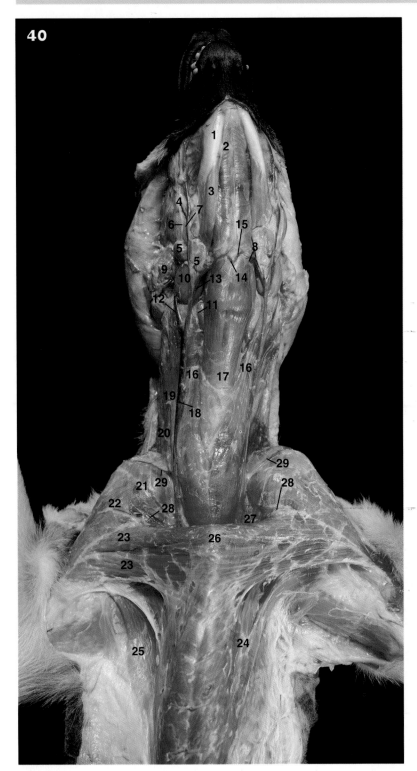

40

1	Body of mandible	16	M. sternomastoideus and
2	M. mylohyoideus		M. sterno-occipitalis
3	M. digastricus		(M. sternocephalicus)
4	M. masseter	17	M. stemohyoideus
5	Mandibular lymph nodes	18	External jugular vein
6	Parotid duct	19	M. cleidomastoideus
7	Facial vein	20	M. cleidocervicalis
8	M. stylohyoideus	21	Clavicular tendon
9	Parotid gland	22	M. cleidobrachialis
10	Mandibular salivary		(M. brachiocephalicus)
	gland	23	Mm. pectorales superficiales
11	Medial retropharyngeal	24	M. pectoralis profundus
	lymph node	25	M. latissimus dorsi
12	Maxillary vein	26	Manubrium sterni
13	Lingual vein	27	Supraclavicular fossa
14	Hyoid venous arch	28	Cephalic vein
15	Submental vein	29	Omobrachial vein

Clinical Note

17   Note the presence of the midline fibrous raphe between the muscles of both sides. Surgical incisions in the cervical region are always made exactly midline ventrally through this raphe to minimise trauma to surrounding tissue and reduce haemorrhage. The muscles can then be spread laterally to reveal deeper structures.

18   The jugular vein, as it runs in this ventrolateral position, is accessible for venepuncture in the conscious dog, being a convenient site for the collection of larger volume blood samples. Blood is flowing towards the thorax and so pressure is placed on the vein at the more caudal ventral cervical region to raise the pressure and engorge the vein prior to insertion of the needle.

41   **Ventral aspect of the head and neck of a dog. The
sternohyoideus and sternothyroideus muscles have been
resected to expose the trachea.**

1	Body of mandible	6	M. thyrohyoideus
2	M. mylohyoideus	7	M. sternothyroideus
3	M. digastricus	8	Thyroid cartilage
4	M. geniohyoideus	9	Cricoid cartilage
5	M. styloglossus	10	Trachea

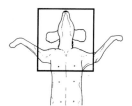

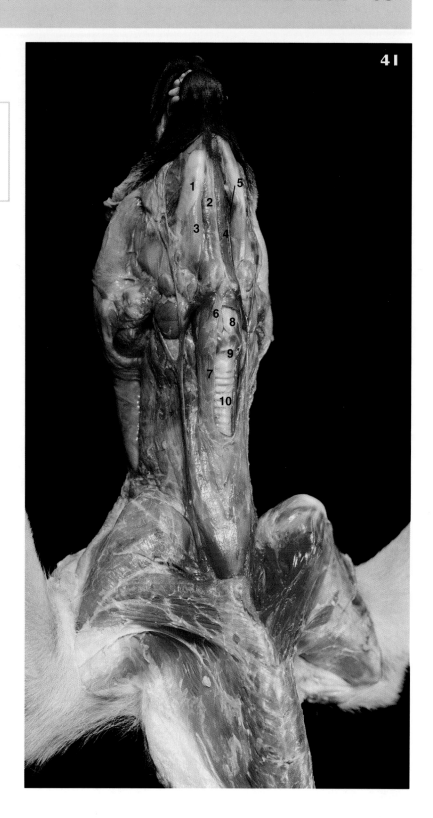

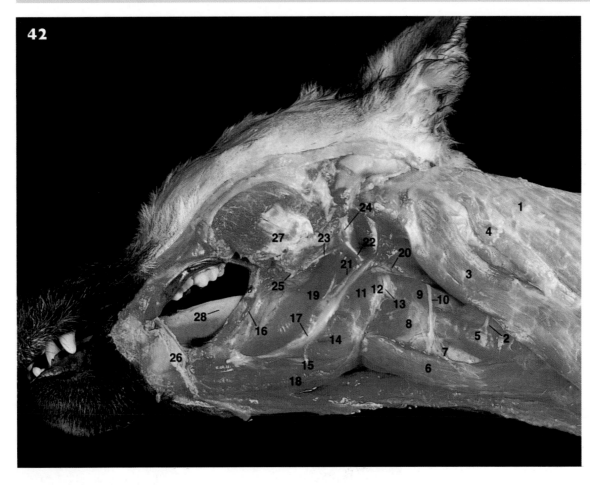

42 Ventrolateral aspect of the muscles of the head and neck of a dog. The left ramus and body of the mandible have been removed by sectioning off the muscles close to their insertions on these structures.

1	M. cleidocervicalis
2	Second cervical nerve
3	M. sternomastoideus ⎱ M. sterno-
4	M. sterno-occipitalis ⎰ cephalicus
5	M. sternothyroideus
6	M. sternohyoideus
7	M. cricothyroideus
8	M. thyrohyoideus
9	M. thyropharyngeus
10	Cervical nerve
11	M. ceratopharyngeus
12	M. chondropharyngeus
13	Cranial laryngeal nerve
14	M. hyoglossus
15	M. geniohyoideus
16	Buccal nerve
17	Hypoglossal nerve
18	M. mylohyoideus
19	M. styloglossus
20	Vagosympathetic trunk
21	Lingual artery
22	External carotid artery
23	Facial artery
24	Maxillary artery
25	Lingual nerve (cut ends)
26	Body of mandible (cut)
27	M. masseter
28	Tongue (folliate papillae)

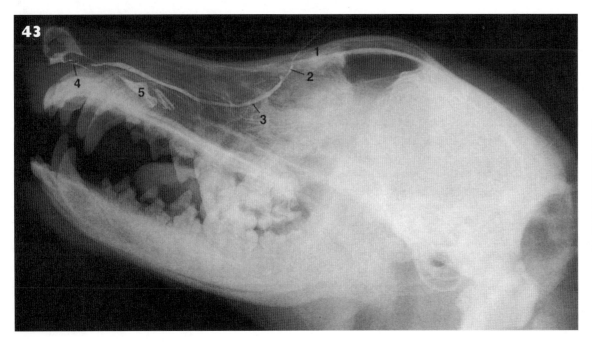

43 Lateral radiograph of the head of a dog. Radio-opaque material has been injected into the ventral lacrimal punctum to demonstrate the course of the nasolacrimal duct.

1	Needle in ventral lacrimal punctum
2	Lacrimal sac
3	Nasolacrimal duct
4	Duct discharging into floor of nasal vestibule
5	Refluxed radio-opaque material in ventral meatus

44 **Rostral aspect of a transverse section of the skull of a dog, at the level of the fourth upper premolar tooth.**

1	Ethmoid bone	7	Vomer
2	Labyrinth (conchae)	8	Choana leading to
3	Perpendicular plate or lamina		nasopharyngeal meatus
4	Lateral lamina	9	Infraorbital canal
5	Maxillary recess	10	Nasolacrimal canal
6	Transverse lamina		

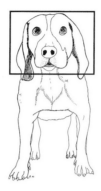

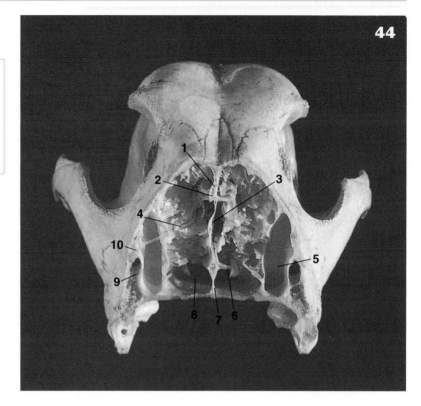

45 **Transverse sections through the nasal cavity of a dog, at the level of (A) the upper canine tooth and (B) the fourth upper premolar tooth.**

Clinical Note

26 Note that the root of this tooth lies immediately ventral to the maxillary recess (**23**). Infection of the tooth root can erode into the recess. If left untreated this can cause swelling in the facial region ventral to the eye and eventually will fistulate through to the exterior, producing a purulent discharge.

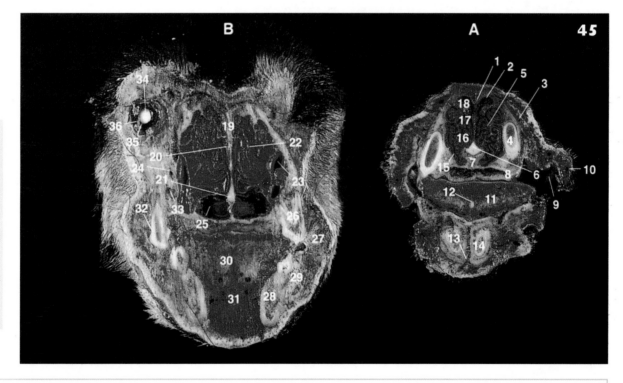

1	Nasal bone	12	Lyssa
2	Dorsal nasal concha	13	Body of mandible
3	Maxilla	14	Lower canine tooth
4	Upper canine tooth	15	Ventral meatus
5	Ventral nasal concha	16	Common meatus
6	Cartilaginous nasal septum	17	Middle meatus
7	Vomer	18	Dorsal meatus
8	Hard palate	19	Septal process of frontal
9	Buccal cavity		bones
10	Upper lip (labia superior)	20	Perpendicular plate, ethmoid
11	Tongue		bone

21	Vomer
22	Ethmoidal conchae
23	Maxillary recess
24	Nasolacrimal duct
25	Nasopharynx
26	Fourth premolar tooth
27	M. buccinator
28	Body of mandible
29	Lower premolar tooth
30	Tongue
31	M. geniohyoideus

32	Root canal of upper molar tooth
33	Infraorbital canal
34	Lens
35	Iris
36	Pupil

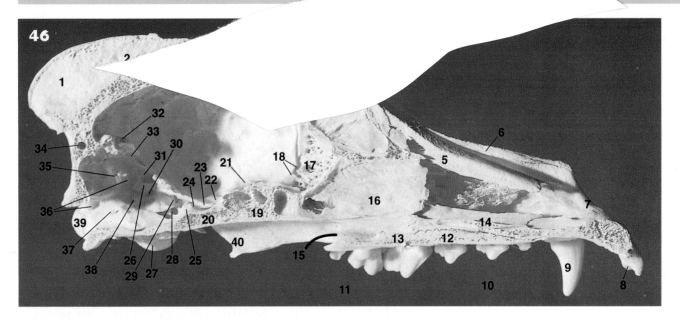

46   Median section of the skull of a dog.

1 Interparietal bone	12 Palatine process of maxilla	20 Body of basisphenoid bone	30 Internal acoustic meatus
2 Parietal bone	13 Horizontal plate of palatine	21 Optical canal	31 Cerebellar fossa
3 Frontal bone	bone	22 Orbital fissure	32 Tentorium osseum
4 Median septum of frontal sinus	14 Vomer	23 Foramen rotundum viewed	33 Transverse groove
5 Nasal bone	15 Nasopharyngeal meatus	through rostral alar foramen	34 Transverse canal
6 Maxilla	16 Osseous nasal septum of eth-	24 Foramen ovale	35 Supramastoid foramen
7 Incisive bone	moid bone	25 Dorsum sellae	36 Condyloid canal
8 Incisor teeth	17 Cribriform plate of ethmoid	26 Petrosal ⎫ part of	37 Hypoglossal canal
9 Canine tooth	bone with cribriform foramina	27 Tympanic ⎭ temporal bone	38 Jugular foramen
10 Premolar teeth	18 Ethmoidal foramina	28 Internal carotid foramen	39 Occipital bone
11 Molar teeth	19 Body of presphenoid bone	29 Canal for the trigeminal nerve	40 Pterygoid bone

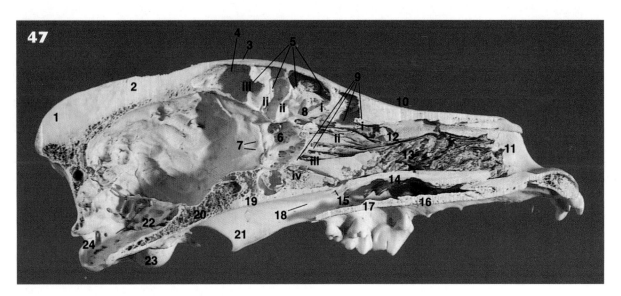

47   Paramedian section of the skull of a dog.

1 Interparietal bone	7 Ethmoidal foramina	13 Ventral nasal conchae	19 Body of presphenoid bone
2 Parietal bone	8 Dorsal lamina	14 Entrance to maxillary recess	20 Body of basisphenoid bone
3 Frontal bone	9 Endoturbinates (i–iv)	15 Sphenopalatine foramen	21 Pterygoid bone
4 Frontal sinus	10 Nasal bone	16 Palatine process of maxilla	22 Petrosal ⎫ part of
5 Ectoturbinates (i–iii)	11 Incisive bone	17 Horizontal plate of palatine bone	23 Tympanic ⎭ temporal bone
6 Cribriform plate	12 Dorsal nasal conchae	18 Nasopharyngeal meatus	24 Occipital bone

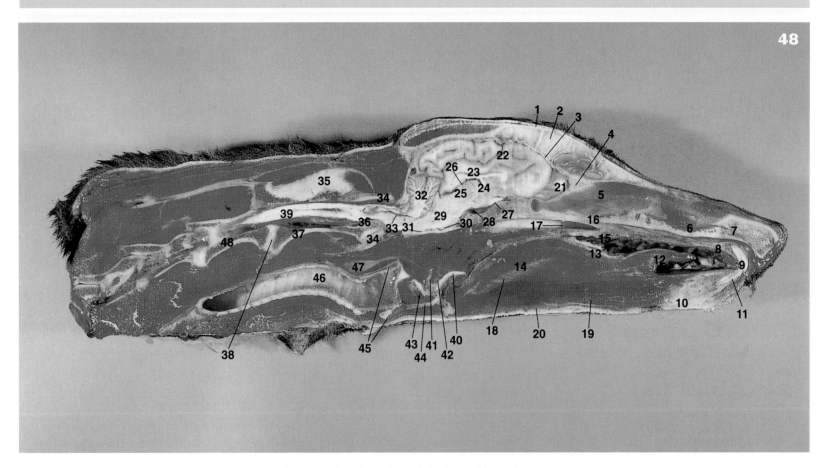

48 Median section of the head and neck of a dog, showing the left half of this region.

1 Frontal bone	26 Thalamus
2 Frontal sinus	27 Optic chiasma
3 Median septum	28 Site of hypophysis cerebri
4 Ethmoid bone	29 Pons
5 Osseous nasal septum	30 Transverse fibres of 29
6 Membranous septum	31 Medulla oblongata
7 Cartilaginous septum	32 Cerebellum
8 Incisive bone	33 Fourth ventricle
9 Upper incisor tooth	34 First cervical vertebra (atlas)
10 Mandible	35 Spinous process ⎱ of second cervical
11 Lower incisor tooth	36 Dens (odontoid process) ⎰ vertebra (axis)
12 Apex ⎱	37 Body of axis
13 Dorsum ⎰ of tongue	38 Intervertebral disc with annulus fibrosus and inner
14 Body ⎱	nucleus pulposus
15 Hard palate ⎰	39 Spinal cord
16 Vomer	40 Epiglottis
17 Choana	41 Arytenoid cartilage
18 M. genioglossus	42 Aditus laryngis
19 M. geniohyoideus	43 Site of lateral ventricle
20 M. mylohyoideus	44 Thyroid cartilage
21 Olfactory bulb	45 Cricoid cartilage
22 Cerebral hemisphere	48 Trachea
23 Corpus callosum	47 Oesophagus
24 Third ventricle	48 Third cervical vertebra
25 Interthalamic adhesion	

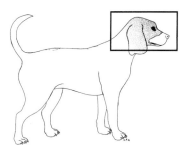

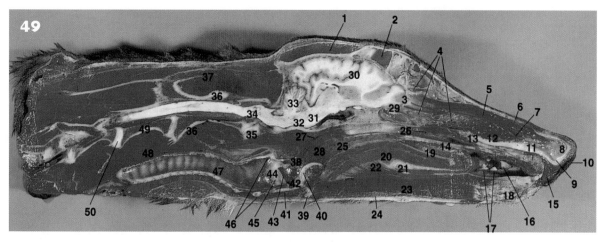

49   Paramedian section of the head and neck of a dog.

Clinical Note
40 Note the relative positions of the epiglottis and the caudal edge of the soft palate. The epiglottis lies dorsal to the soft palate simulating the situation found during nasal breathing. To introduce an endotracheal tube via the oral cavity with the intention of entering the larynx and trachea in an anaesthetised dog would require that the soft palate be elevated dorsal to the epiglottis and then the tube could enter the aditus laryngis.

1 M. temporalis	18 Mandible	35 First cervical vertebra (atlas)
2 Frontal sinus	19 Apex (reflected caudally)	36 Second cervical vertebra (axis)
3 Cribriform plate of ethmoid bone	20 Body } of tongue	37 M. rectus capitis dorsalis
4 Ethmoidal conchae	21 Lyssa	38 Laryngopharynx
5 Dorsal nasal concha	22 M. genioglossus	39 Hyoid bone
6 Dorsal meatus	23 M. geniohyoideus	40 Epiglottis
7 Middle meatus	24 M. mylohyoideus	41 Thyroid cartilage
8 Alar fold	25 Soft palate	42 Vestibular fold
9 Cartilage of nasal septum	26 Choana	43 Lateral ventricle
10 External nares (nostrils)	27 Opening of auditory tube	44 Vocal process of arytenoid cartilage
11 Ventral meatus	28 Nasopharynx	45 Vocal fold
12 Ventral nasal concha	29 Olfactory bulb	48 Cricoid cartilage
13 Vomer	30 Cerebral hemisphere	47 Trachea
14 Hard palate	31 Pons	48 M. longus colli
15 Upper lip (labia superior)	32 Medulla oblongata	49 Body of third cervical vertebra
16 Canine teeth	33 Cerebellum	50 Intervertebral disc with outer annulus fibrosus and inner nucleus pulposus
17 Premolar teeth	34 Spinal cord	

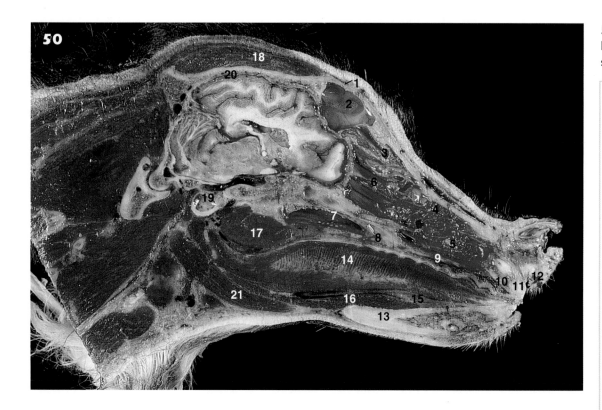

50   Paramedian section of the head of a dog revealing the structures of the left nasal cavity.

1	Frontal bone
2	Lateral part of frontal sinus
3	Ethmoidal conchae
4	Dorsal nasal conchae
5	Ventral nasal conchae
6	Lateral lamina of ethmoid bone
7	Choana
8	Palatine bone
9	Maxilla
10	Incisive bone
11	Upper incisor tooth
12	Upper lip (labia superior)
13	Mandible
14	Body of tongue
15	M. genioglossus
16	M. geniohyoideus
17	M. pterygoideus medialis
18	M. temporalis
19	Temporal bone
20	Parietal bone
21	M. digastricus

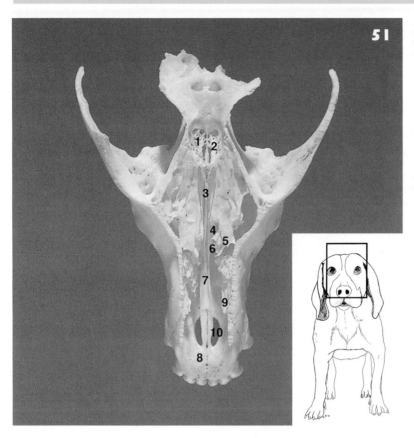

51 Nasal region of the skull of a dog, sectioned in the dorsal plane.

1	Ethmoid bone	6	Horizontal ⎱ part of vomer
2	Cribriform plate	7	Sagittal ⎰
3	Perpendicular plate or lamina	8	Incisive bone
4	Transverse lamina	9	Ventral nasal conchae
5	Endoturbinates	10	Palatine fissure

52 Dorsal aspect of a coronal section through the head of a dog, at the level of the bony orbit, revealing the contents of the nasal cavity. The section has been made in the dorsal plane.

1	M. temporalis	13	Nares (nostrils)
2	Cerebral hemispheres	14	Maxilla
3	Olfactory bulbs	15	Lacrimal sac
4	Cribriform plate ⎱ of	16	Cornea
5	Perpendicular ⎰ ethmoid	17	Anterior chamber
	plate ⎰ bone	18	Iris
6	Dorsal nasal conchae	19	Posterior chamber
7	Ethmoidal conchae	20	Pupil
8	Median septum	21	Ciliary body
9	Cartilaginous septum	22	Lens
10	Alar fold	23	Vitreous chamber
11	Nasal vestibule	24	Fundus
12	Opening of nasolacrimal duct	25	Orbit

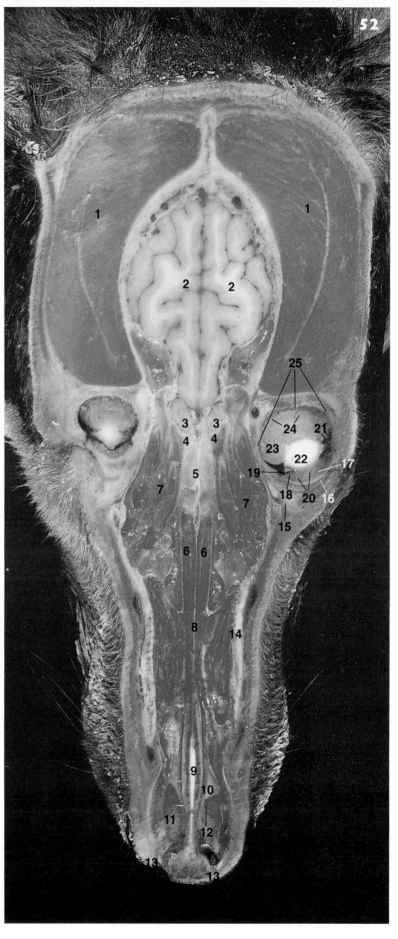

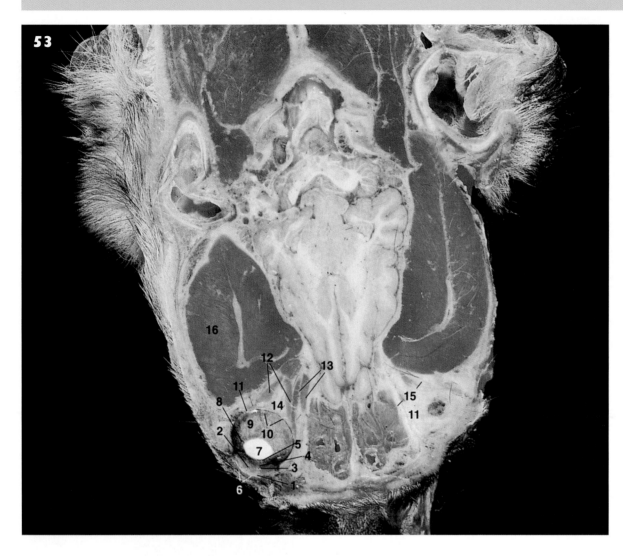

53

53 Dorsal aspect of an oblique section in the dorsal plane, made through the head of a dog at the level of the orbit. The structure of the eyeball and the orbital contents are shown.

1	Bulbar conjunctiva covering cornea
2	Cornea
3	Anterior chamber
4	Iris
5	Posterior chamber
6	Pupil
7	Lens
8	Ciliary body
9	Vitreous chamber
10	Fundus
11	Sclera
12	M. retractor bulbi
13	Mm. recti
14	Optic nerve
15	Periorbita
16	M. temporalis

54

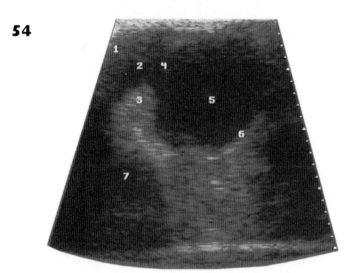

54 Ultrasound scan of the eye of a dog, demonstrating the contents of the bulb of the eye. The healthy lens is almost echolucent, but its position is marked (4). The plane of the scan is horizontal and corresponds to Fig. 53.

1	Corneal surface	5	Vitreous chamber
2	Anterior chamber	6	Caudal scleral surface (with
3	Ciliary body		retrobulbar contents distal to it)
4	Lens	7	Medial aspect of orbit

55 Lateral aspect of a sagittal section through the head of a dog. The structure of the eyeball and the orbital contents are shown.

 1 Upper eyelid (palpebra superior)
 2 Medial commissure
 3 Frontal bone
 4 Conjunctival sac
 5 Cornea
 6 Anterior chamber
 7 Ciliary body
 8 Lens
 9 Vitreous chamber
10 Retinal layer
11 Choroid
12 Mm. recti
13 M. retractor bulbi
14 M. obliquus ventralis
15 Zygomatic gland
16 Maxilla
17 Upper molar teeth
18 M. temporalis
19 M. pterygoideus
20 Tongue
21 Larynx

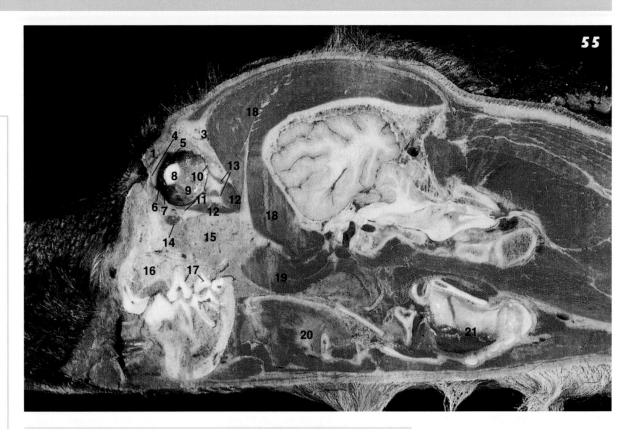

Clinical Note
This section of the head gives an anatomical plane similar to that in a vertical ultrasound scan of the eye.

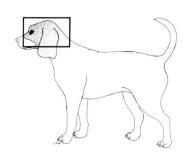

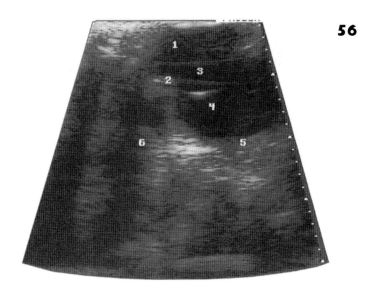

56 Ultrasound scan of the eye of a dog, demonstrating the contents of the bulb of the eye (eyeball). The plane of the scan is vertical and corresponds to Fig. 55. The caudal surface of the lens is indicated by a white line between 3 and 4, which is due to specular reflection from the lens surface.

1 Anterior chamber	4 Vitreous chamber	
2 Ciliary body	5 Optic disc region	
3 Lens	6 Ventral aspect of the orbit	

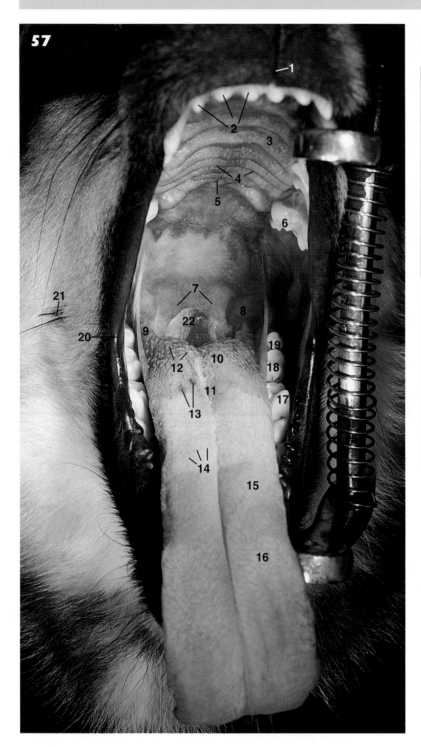

57   Rostral aspect of the open oral cavity, revealing the structures of the caudal oral cavity

1	Philtrum	12	Filiform papillae
2	Upper incisor teeth	13	Vallate papillae
3	Hard palate	14	Fungiform papillae
4	Palatine ridges	15	Body ⎤ of tongue
5	Palatine raphe	16	Dorsal face ⎦
6	Fourth upper premolar	17	First ⎤
	(carnassial) tooth	18	Second ⎬ lower molar tooth
7	Soft palate	19	Third ⎦
8	Palatine tonsils in crypt	20	Angle of mouth
9	Palatoglossal arch	21	Vibrissae
10	Root of tongue	22	Epiglottis
11	Median groove		

Clinical Note

7   Note that the soft palate lies dorsal to the free edge of the epiglottis, simulating the position found in oral breathing. This is the required relative positioning of the epiglottis and soft palate in order to facilitate the introduction of an endotracheal tube via the oral route.

8   The palatine tonsil is normally obscured by the overlying mucosa of the crypt. During clinical examination an attempt is made to visualise the tonsil which will become enlarged in the infective state and be readily visible bulging from its crypt.

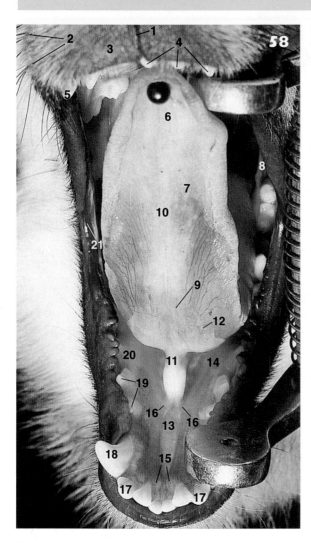

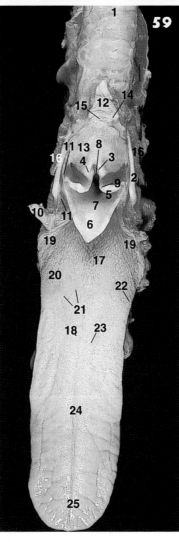

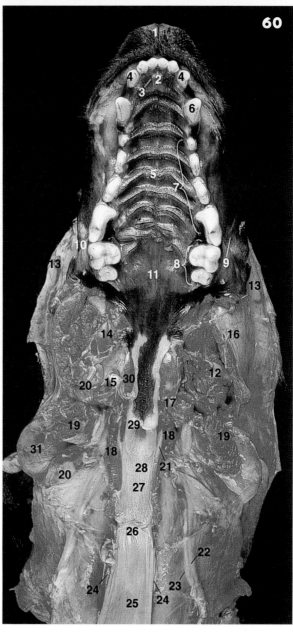

58 Rostral aspect of the oral cavity of a dog. The tongue has been elevated dorsally to reveal the ventral floor of the oral cavity.

59 Dorsal aspect of the tongue and larynx of a dog.

60 Ventral aspect of a section of the head of a dog, made in the dorsal plane through the digestive tube.

1 Philtrum	14 Lateral sublingual
2 Tactile hairs	recess
3 Upper lip (labia	15 Orobasal organ
superior)	16 Sublingual caruncle
4 Upper incisor teeth	with opening of
5 Upper canine tooth	mandibular duct
6 Apex ⎤ of	and major
7 Ventral ⎬ tongue	sublingual duct
face ⎦	17 Lower incisor teeth
8 Buccal vestibule	18 Lower canine tooth
9 Lingual vein	19 First and second
10 Position of lyssa	lower premolar
11 Sublingual frenulum	teeth
12 Fimbriated plica	20 Gums
13 Sublingual recess	21 Angle of mouth

1 Trachea	
2 Dorsal border of thyroid	
cartilage	
3 Corniculate process of	
arytenoid cartilage	
4 Corniculate ⎤	
5 Cuneiform ⎦ tubercle	
7 Laryngeal inlet	
8 Interarytenoid groove	
9 Aryepiglottic fold	
10 Hyoid bone	
11 Piriform recess	
12 Oesophagus	
13 Caudal part of	
laryngopharynx	
14 Pharyngo-oesophageal	
junction	
15 Limen pharyngoesophageum	
16 Palatopharyngeal arch	
17 Root ⎤ of tongue	
18 Body ⎦	
19 Palatopharyngeal arch	
20 Filiform papillae	
21 Vallate papillae	
22 Foliate papillae	
23 Fungiform papillae	
24 Median groove (sulcus)	
25 Apex of tongue	

1	Philtrum	18	Pharyngeal muscles
2	Incisive papilla	19	M. digastricus
3	Orifice of incisive	20	Mandibular lymph
	duct		mode
4	Incisor teeth	21	Thyroid cartilage
5	Hard palate	22	Common carotid
6	Canine teeth		artery
7	Premolar teeth	23	Vagosympathetic
8	Molar teeth		trunk
9	Orifice of parotid	24	Thyroid gland
	duct	25	Oesophagus
10	Region of orifices of	26	Annular fold
	zygomatic ducts	27	Dorsal wall of
11	Soft palate		laryngeal pharynx
12	Mandible	28	Pharyngeal isthmus
13	M. buccinator	29	Pharyngopalatine
14	M. styloglossus		arch
15	Epihyoid bone	30	Palatine tonsil
16	M. masseter	31	Mandibular salivary
17	Hypoglossal nerve		gland

Clinical Note

16 In clinical cases where it is suspected that there is an occlusion of the ducts of either the mandibular or the monostomatic sublingual salivary glands, the caruncle is identified and the duct openings cannulated in order to introduce radio-opaque material to discover the patency of the ducts. Example of such a radiograph are shown in Figs 61 and 62.

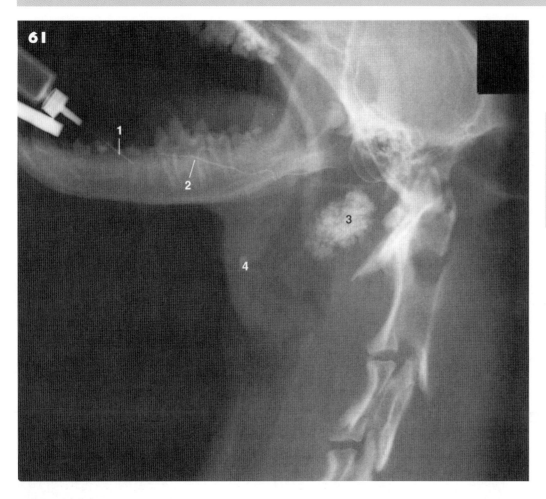

61   Lateral radiograph of the head of a dog. To demonstrate the position of the mandibular salivary gland, radio-opaque material has been injected into the duct of the gland.

1 Needle inserted into orifice of duct of mandibular salivary gland at sublingual caruncle
2 Duct of mandibular salivary gland
3 Mandibular salivary gland
4 Hyoid bone

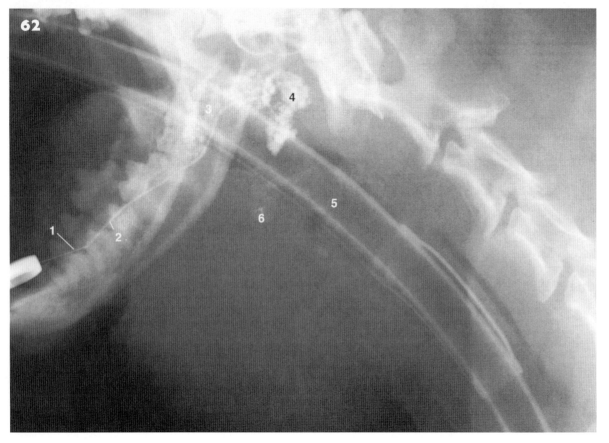

62   Lateral radiograph of the head of a dog. Radio-opaque material has been injected into the duct of the monostomatic sublingual salivary gland to outline its course and the glandular tissue.

1 Needle inserted into orifice of duct of monostomatic sublingual salivary gland at sublingual caruncle
2 Duct of monostomatic sublingual salivary gland
3 Glandular tissue around duct
4 Portion of monostomatic sublingual salivary gland encapsulated with mandibular salivary gland
5 Endotracheal tube
6 Hyoid bone

63 Cranial aspect of the first (atlas) (A), second (axis) (B), and fifth cervical vertebrae (C) of a dog.

1 Dorsal tubercle
2 Lateral vertebral foramen
3 Transverse foramen
4 Cranial articular fovea
5 Transverse process (wing of atlas)
6 Body
7 Ventral tubercle
8 Dorsal arch
9 Spinous process
10 Caudal articular process
11 Cranial articular surface
12 Dens (odontoid process)
13 Transverse canal
14 Lamina
15 Vertebral foramen

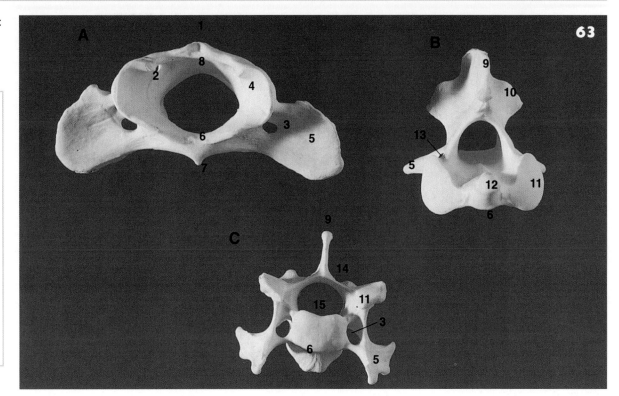

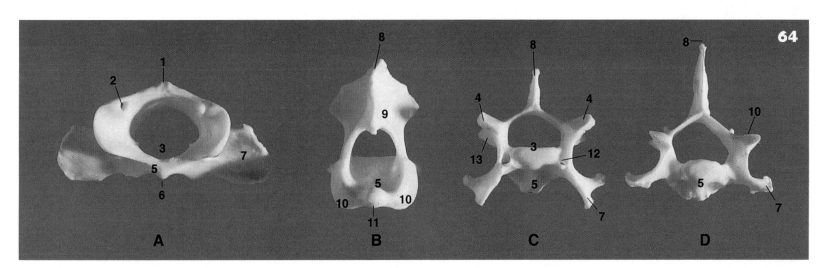

64 Cranial aspect of the first (atlas) (A), second (axis) (B), fifth (C) and seventh cervical vertebrae (D) of a cat.

1 Dorsal tubercle	6 Ventral tubercle	10 Cranial articular surface
2 Lateral vertebral foramen	7 Transverse process (wing of atlas)	11 Dens (odontoid process)
3 Vertebral foramen		12 Transverse foramen
4 Cranial articular fovea	8 Spinous process	13 Caudal articular process
5 Body	9 Arch	

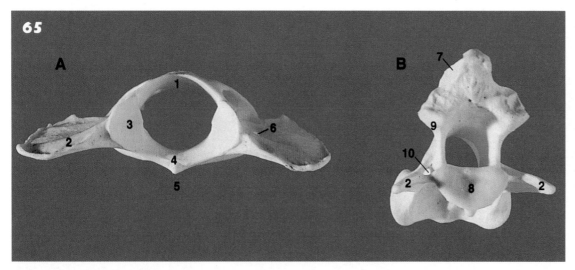

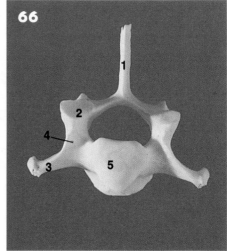

65   Caudal aspect of the first (atlas) (A) and second (axis) (B) cervical vertebrae of a dog.

1 Arch	6 Transverse foramen
2 Transverse process	7 Spinous process
3 Caudal articular fovea	8 Body of axis
4 Fovea for dens (odontoid process)	9 Caudal articular process
	10 Transverse foramen
5 Ventral tubercle	

66   Cranial aspect of the seventh cervical vertebra of a dog.

1 Spinous process
2 Cranial articular surface
3 Transverse process
4 Transverse foramen
5 Body

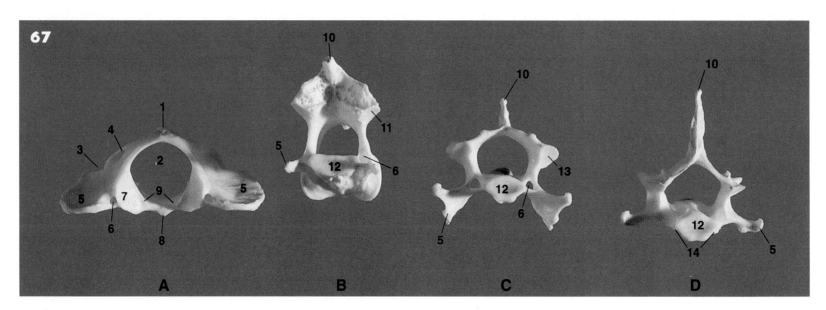

67   Caudal aspect of the first (atlas) (A), second (axis) (B), fifth (C) and seventh cervical vertebrae (D) of a cat.

1 Dorsal tubercle	6 Transverse foramen	11 Caudal articular surface
2 Vertebral foramen	7 Caudal articular fovea	12 Body
3 Alar notch	8 Ventral tubercle	13 Caudal articular surface
4 Lateral vertebral foramen	9 Fovea of dens	14 Caudal costal fovea
5 Transverse process	10 Spinous process	

68   Ventral aspect of the first (atlas) and second (axis) cervical vertebrae of a cat.

1	Atlas	7	Atlantoaxial articulation
2	Axis	8	Ventral tubercle
3	Cranial articular fovea	9	Body
4	Dens (odontoid process)	10	Transverse process
5	Wing of atlas	11	Caudal articular surface
6	Transverse foramen		

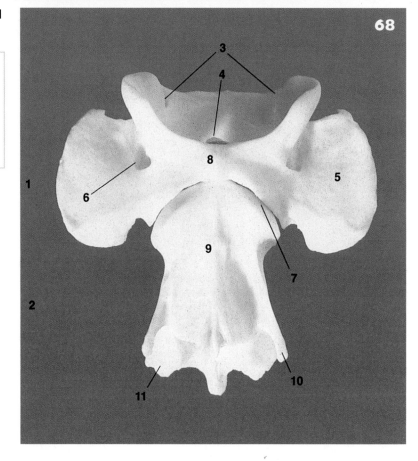

69   Dorsal aspect of the first (A) (atlas), second (axis) (B), and third (C) cervical vertebrae of a cat.

1	Lateral vertebral foramen	4	Spinous process
2	Alar notch	5	Atlantoaxial articulation
3	Transverse process	6	Caudal articular process

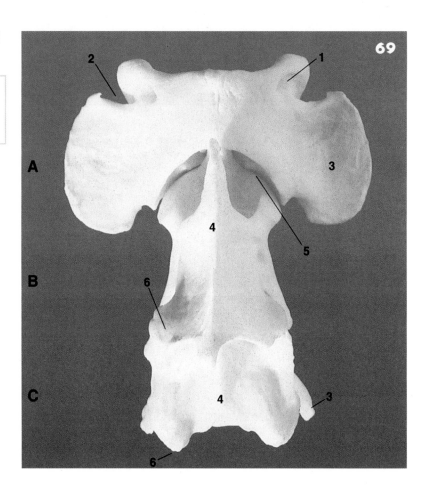

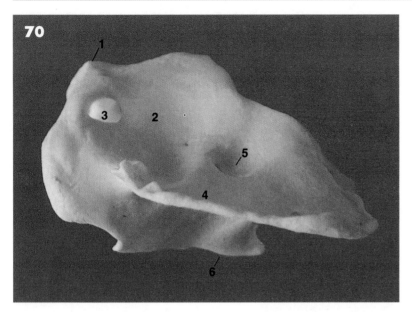

70   Lateral aspect of the first cervical vertebra (atlas) of a dog.

1 Dorsal tubercle	5 Transverse foramen
2 Arch	6 Ventral tubercle
3 Lateral vertebral foramen	
4 Transverse process (wing of atlas)	

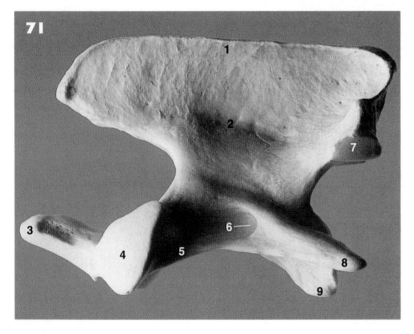

71   Lateral aspect of the second cervical vertebra (axis) of a dog.

1 Spinous process	6 Transverse foramen
2 Arch	7 Caudal articular process
3 Dens (odontoid process)	8 Transverse process
4 Cranial articular surface	9 Median ventral crest
5 Body	

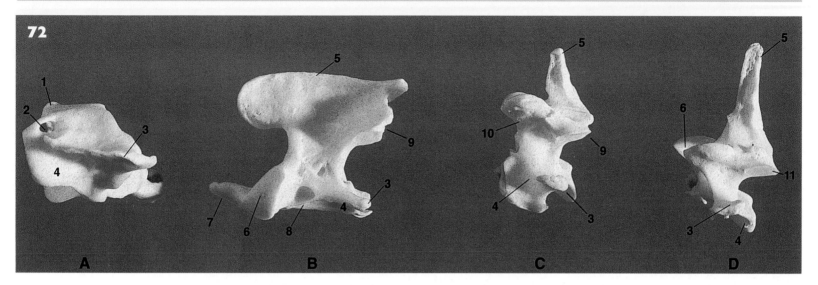

72   Left lateral aspect of the first (atlas) (A), second (axis) (B), fifth (C) and seventh (D) cervical vertebrae of a cat.

1 Dorsal tubercle	5 Spinous process	9 Caudal articular process
2 Lateral vertebral foramen	6 Cranial articular surface	10 Cranial articular process
3 Transverse process	7 Dens (odontoid process)	11 Caudal articular surface
4 Body	8 Transverse foramen	

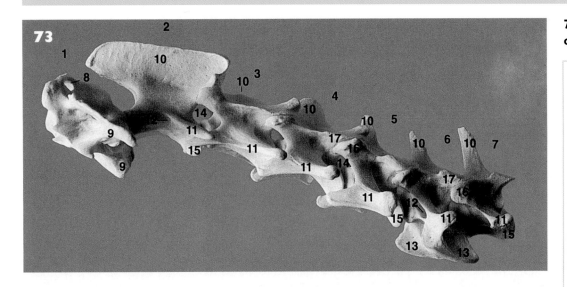

73   Lateral aspect of the articulated cervical vertebrae of a dog.

1	First (atlas)	
2	Second (axis)	
3	Third	
4	Fourth	cervical
5	Fifth	vertebrae
6	Sixth	
7	Seventh	
8	Lateral vertebral foramen	
9	Wing of 1	
10	Spinous process	
11	Transverse process	
12	Transverse foramen	
13	Expanded plate of transverse process of 6	
14	Intervertebral foramen	
15	Body	
16	Cranial articular process	
17	Caudal articular process	

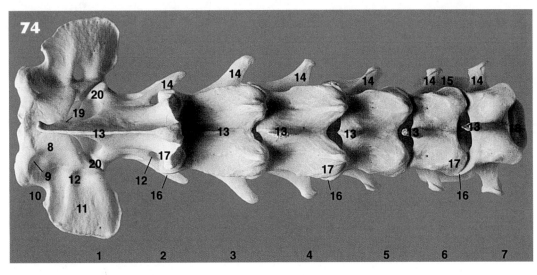

74   Dorsal aspect of the articulated cervical vertebrae of a dog.

1	First (atlas)		8	Arch	15	Expanded plate of	
2	Second (axis)		9	Lateral vertebral foramen		transverse process of 6	
3	Third	cervical	10	Alar notch	16	Cranial articular process	
4	Fourth	vertebrae	11	Wing of 1	17	Caudal articular process	
5	Fifth		12	Transverse foramen	18	Body	
6	Sixth		13	Spinous process	19	Dens	
7	Seventh		14	Transverse process	20	Atlantoaxial articulation	

75   Ventral aspect of the articulated cervical vertebrae of a dog.

1	First (atlas)	
2	Second (axis)	
3	Third	
4	Fourth	cervical vertebrae
5	Fifth	
6	Sixth	
7	Seventh	
8	Body	
9	Wing	
10	Transverse foramen	
11	Cranial articular fovea	
12	Alar notch	
13	Ventral tubercle	
14	Dens	
15	Atlantoaxial articulation	
16	Transverse process	
17	Expanded plate of transverse process of 6	
18	Cranial articular process	

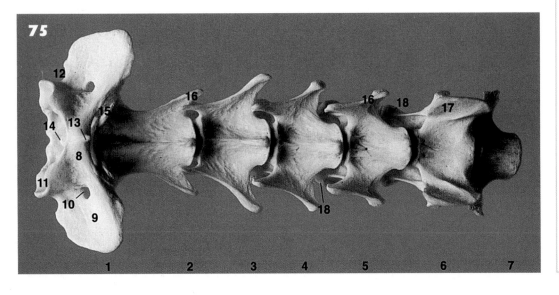
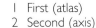

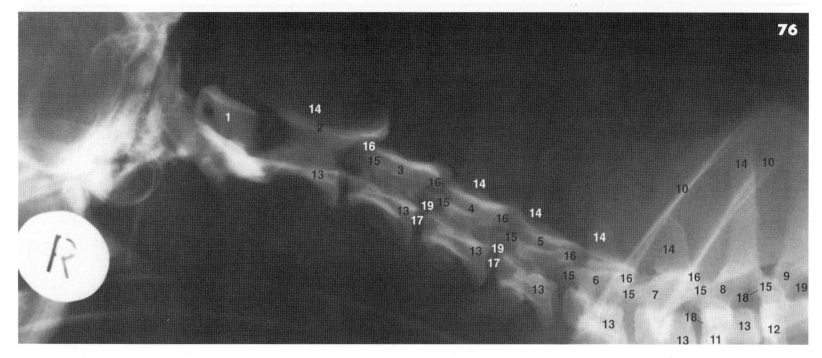

76 Lateral radiograph of the cervical portion of the vertebral column of a dog.

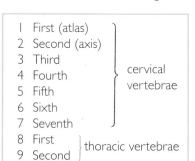

I	First (atlas)
2	Second (axis)
3	Third
4	Fourth
5	Fifth
6	Sixth
7	Seventh
8	First
9	Second
I0	Scapula
II	First
I2	Second
I3	Body
I4	Spinous process
I5	Cranial articular process
I6	Caudal articular process
I7	Location of intervertebral disc
I8	Fovea for articulation of rib
I9	Intervertebral foramen

3–7 cervical vertebrae
8–9 thoracic vertebrae
11–12 rib

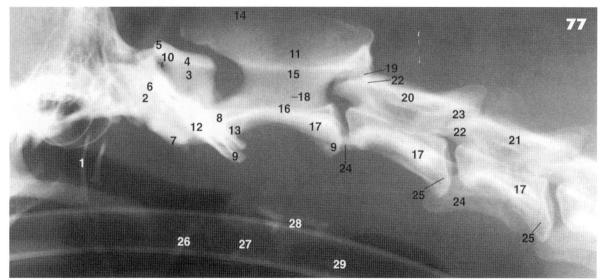

77 Lateral radiograph of the cranial cervical portion of the vertebral column of a dog.

I	Stylohyoid bone	I5	Dorsal border
2	Occipital condyle	I6	Ventral border
3	First cervical vertebra (atlas)	I7	Body
4	Dorsal arch	I8	Transverse foramen
5	Dorsal tubercle	I9	Articular processes
6	Border of cranial articular surface	20	Third
7	Ventral arch	21	Fourth
8	Border of caudal articular surface	22	Cranial articular process
9	Transverse process	23	Caudal articular process
I0	Lateral vertebral foramen	24	Cranial extension
II	Second cervical vertebra (axis)	25	Caudal extension
I2	Dens	26	Thyrohyoid bone
I3	Cranial articular surface	27	Thyroid cartilage
I4	Spinous process	28	Cricoid cartilage
		29	Trachea (with endotracheal tube)

15–16 of vertebral foramen (vertebral canal)
20–21 cervical vertebra
24–25 of transverse process

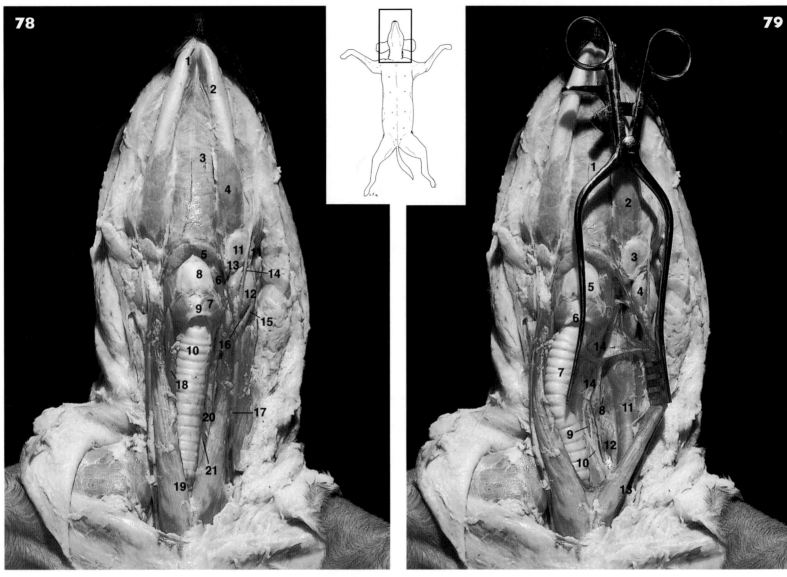

78   Ventral aspect of the deep structures of the neck of a dog. The ventral muscles have been resected to expose the trachea.

1	Mandibular symphysis	13	Lingual vein
2	Mandibular body	14	Facial vein
3	M. mylohyoideus	15	Maxillary vein
4	M. digastricus	16	Linguofacial vein
5	M. sternohyoideus (cut edge)	17	External jugular vein
6	M. thyrohyoideus	18	M. sternothyrohyoideus
7	M. cricothyroideus	19	M. sternocephalicus
8	Thyroid cartilage	20	Carotid sheath with
9	Cricoid cartilage		vagosympathetic trunk, carotid
10	Tracheal rings		artery and internal jugular
11	Mandibular lymph nodes		vein
12	Mandibular salivary gland	21	Recurrent laryngeal nerve

Clinical Note

18   This view simulates the appearance of a midline ventral surgical approach to the cervical region. The median raphe between the Mm. sternothyrohyoideus is split and the muscles divided to reveal the deeper structures.

79   Ventral aspect of the deep structures of the neck of a dog. The trachea has been deviated from the midline to reveal the oesophagus and carotid sheath.

1	M. mylohyoideus	8	Carotid artery
2	M. digastricus	9	Vagosympathetic trunk
3	Mandibular lymph node	10	Recurrent laryngeal nerve
4	Mandibular salivary gland	11	Oesophagus
5	Thyroid cartilage	12	M. longus colli
6	Cricoid cartilage	13	M. sternocephalicus
7	Trachea diverted to right	14	Thyroid gland

Clinical Note

11   This view simulates the appearance of a midline ventral approach to the cervical region used for such purposes as oesophagotomy or cervical disc fenestration. Care must be taken when manipulating the oesophagus to identify and preserve the left recurrent laryngeal nerve (**10**) which lies between the oesophagus and the trachea on the left of the midline

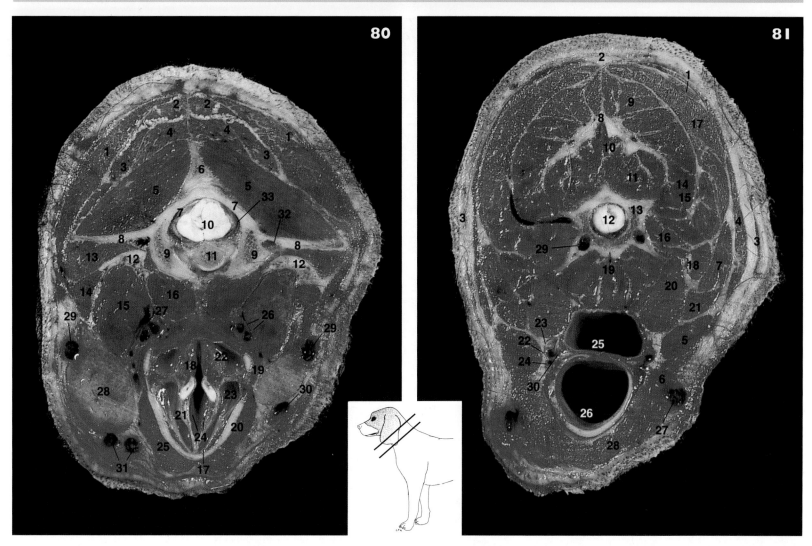

80 Cranial aspect of a transverse section through the neck of a dog at the level of the atlantoaxial joint.

81 Cranial aspect of a transverse section through the neck of a dog at the level of the third cervical vertebra.

1	M. splenius capitis	16	M. rectus capitis ventralis
2	M. semispinalis capitis (biventer)	17	Larynx
3	M. semispinalis capitis (complexus)	18	Arytenoid cartilages
		19	Cricoid cartilage
4	M. rectus capitis dorsalis major	20	Thyroid cartilage
		21	Vocal folds
5	M. obliquus capitis caudalis	22	M. cricoarytenoideus dorsalis
6	Spinous process of second cervical vertebra (axis)	23	Lateral ventricle
		24	Rima glottis
7	Arch	of first cervical	25	M. thyrohyoideus
8	Wing	vertebra (atlas)	26	Division of common carotid artery into external and internal carotid arteries
9	Body		
10	Spinal cord		
11	Dens (odontoid process) of second cervical vertebra (axis)	27	Vagosympathetic trunk
		28	Mandibular salivary gland
		29	Maxillary vein
12	Jugular process	30	Linguofacial vein
13	Mm. intertransversarii cervicis	31	Linguofacial and facial veins (divided)
14	M. omotransversarius	32	Vertebral artery and vein
15	M. longus capitis	33	Internal vertebral plexus

1	M. rhomboideus capitis	14	Mm. longissimus capitis and atlantis
2	Dorsal median raphe		
3	Mm. cutanei colli	15	M. longissimus cervicis
4	M. brachiocephalicus (M. cleidocephalicus, pars cervicalis)	16	Mm. intertransversarius dorsalis, medius and ventralis
		17	M. splenius
5	M. sternocephalicus, pars occipitalis, and M. cleidocephalicus, pars mastoidea	18	M. serratus ventralis cervicis
		19	M. longus colli
		20	M. longus capitis
		21	M. scalenus medius
6	M. sternocephalicus, pars mastoidea	22	Common carotid artery
		23	Vagosympathetic trunk
7	M. omotransversarius	24	Internal jugular vein
8	Ligamentum nuchae	25	Oesophagus
9	M. semispinalis capitis (biventer and complexus)	26	Trachea
		27	External jugular vein
10	M. multifidus cervicis	28	M. sternohyoideus and M. sternothyroideus
11	M. spinalis cervicis		
12	Spinal cord	29	Vertebral artery and vein
13	Third cervical vertebra	30	Recurrent laryngeal nerve

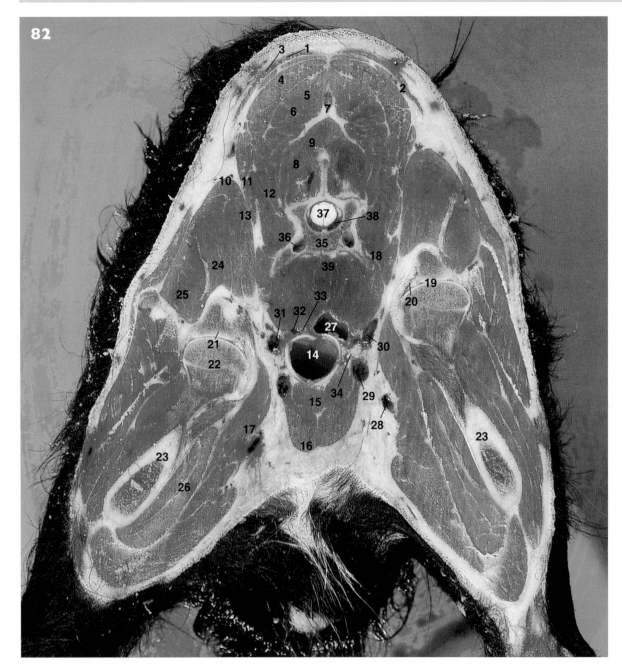

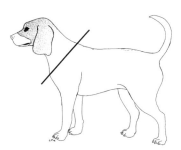

82   **Cranial aspect of a transverse section through the neck of a dog at the level of the seventh cervical vertebra.**

1 M. rhomboideus	14 Trachea	26 M. biceps brachii
2 Mm. cutanei colli	15 M. sternohyoidideus and	27 Oesophagus
3 M. trapezius	M. sternothyroideus	28 Cephalic vein
4 M. splenius	16 M. sternocephalicus	29 Jugular vein
5 M. biventer	17 M. brachiocephalicus	30 Superficial cervical vein
6 M. complexus	(M. cleidobrachialis)	31 Common carotid artery
7 Ligamentum nuchae	18 Mm. intertransversarii	32 Internal jugular vein
8 M. multifidus cervicis	19 Shoulder joint	33 Vagosympathetic trunk
9 M. spinalis cervicis	20 Joint capsule	34 Recurrent laryngeal nerve
10 M. serratus ventralis cervicis	21 Glenoid surface of scapula	35 Seventh cervical vertebra
11 M. longissimus cervicis	22 Head } of humerus	36 Vertebral artery and vein
12 Mm. longissimus capitis and	23 Body	37 Spinal cord
atlantis	24 M. supraspinatus	38 Internal vertebral plexus
13 M. omotransversarius	25 M. infraspinatus	39 M. longus colli

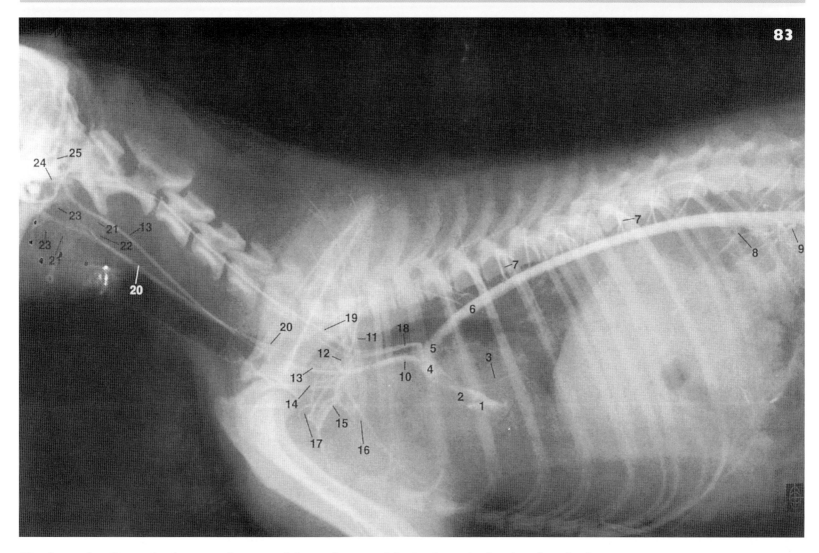

83   Lateral radiograph of an arteriogram of the major arterial vessels to the head and neck of a dog.

1	Left ventricular outflow tract	10	Brachiocephalic trunk	19	Left vertebral artery
2	Aortic valve	11	Right costocervical trunk	20	Left common carotid artery
3	Coronary artery	12	Right vertebral artery	21	Cranial laryngeal artery
4	Ascending aorta	13	Right common carotid artery	22	Internal carotid artery
5	Aortic arch	14	Right subclavian artery	23	Lingual artery
6	Descending aorta	15	Axillary artery	24	Facial artery
7	Segmental arteries	16	Internal thoracic artery	25	Maxillary artery
8	Coeliac artery	17	External thoracic artery		
9	Cranial mesenteric artery	18	Left subclavian artery		

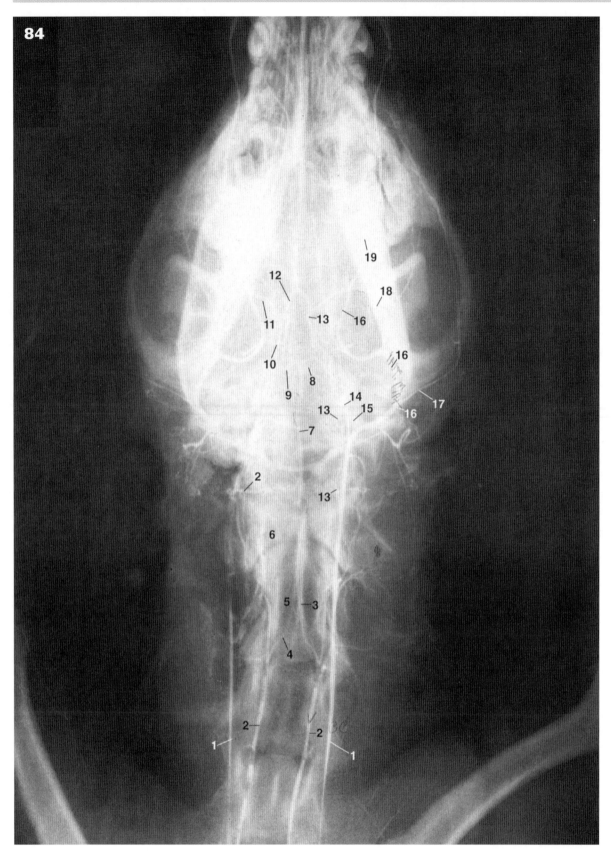

84

1   Common carotid artery
2   Vertebral artery
3   Ventral spinal artery
4   Spinal ramus
5   Second cervical vertebra (axis)
6   First cervical vertebra (atlas)
7   Basilar artery
8   Caudal communicating artery
9   Rostral cerebellar artery
10 Caudal cerebral artery
11 Middle cerebral artery
12 Rostral cerebral artery
13 Internal carotid artery
14 Lingual artery
15 Facial artery
16 Maxillary artery
17 Superficial temporal artery
18 Mandibular alveolar artery
19 Infraorbital artery

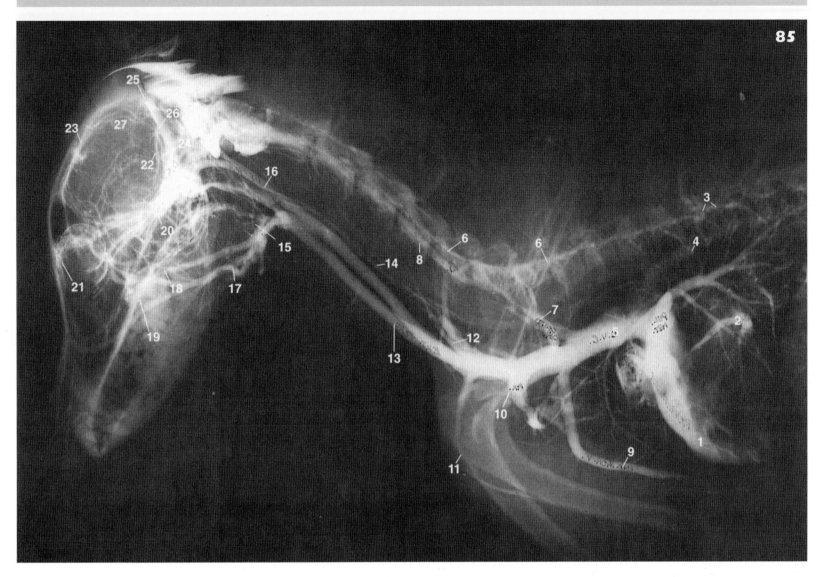

85   Lateral radiograph of a venogram of the head and neck of a dog.

1 Right ventricle	10 Axillary vein	20 Cavernous sinus
2 Coronary veins	11 Cephalic vein	21 Angular vein of eye
3 Intercostal veins	12 Superficial cervical vein	22 Temporal sinus
4 Azygos vein	13 External jugular vein	23 Dorsal sagittal sinus
5 Cranial vena cava	14 Internal jugular vein	24 Straight sinus
6 Internal vertebral venous	15 Linguofacial vein	25 Transverse sinus
plexus	16 Maxillary vein	26 Sigmoid sinus
7 Costocervical vein	17 Lingual vein	27 Dorsal petrosal sinus
8 Vertebral vein	18 Deep facial vein	
9 Internal thoracic vein	19 Facial vein	

3 SPINAL COLUMN

Using bony specimens and radiographs, the osteology of the vertebral column is demonstrated in the other chapters of the book, where such detail is more relevant to the understanding of the anatomy of the respective regions. This short chapter is designed to illustrate the particular muscul-ature surrounding the spinal column, together with the contents of the vertebral canal, by means of fresh dissected material.

86 Lateral aspect of the superficial epaxial muscles and the muscles of the thoracic cage of a dog. The left thoracic limb with its extrinsic muscles has been removed, as has the cutaneous trunci muscle.

  1 M. splenius cervicis
  2 M. longissimus cervicis
  3 M. serratus dorsalis cranialis
  4 M. longissimus thoracis
  5 M. spinalis and M. semispinalis thoracis
  6 Mm. longissimus thoracis and lumborum
  7 M. iliocostalis
  8 Mm. intercostales
  9 M. scalenus
 10 Trachea
 11 M. sternothyroideus
 12 M. sternocephalicus
 13 External jugular vein
 14 Mm. pectorales superficiales (cut)
 15 M. pectoralis profundus (cut)
 16 M. rectus abdominis
 17 M. obliquus externus abdominis
 18 Distal lateral cutaneous branches of intercostal nerves
 19 Manubrium sterni
 20 Costochondral joints
 21 Sternocostal joints

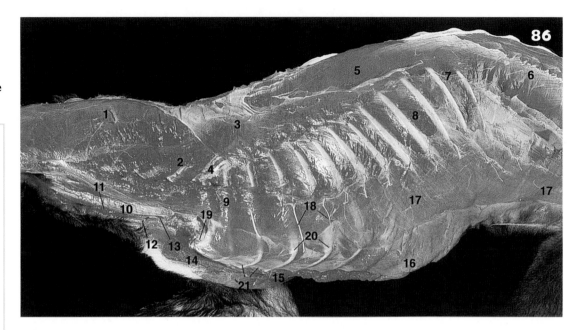

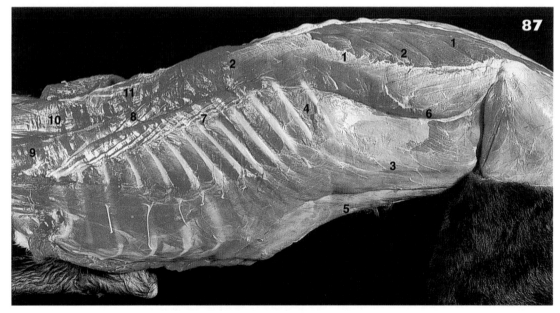

87 Lateral aspect of the deep epaxial muscles of the trunk of a dog. The dorsal serratus cranialis muscle has been removed.

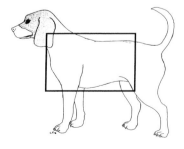

1	Lumbodorsal fascia (cut)	6	M. iliocostalis lumborum
2	Mm. longissimus thoracis and lumborum	7	M. iliocostalis thoracis
3	M. obliquus externus abdominis	8	M. longissimus cervicis
4	M. obliquus internus abdominis	9	M. spinalis capitis
5	M. rectus abdominis	10	M. semispinalis capitis
		11	M. spinalis and M. semispinalis thoracis

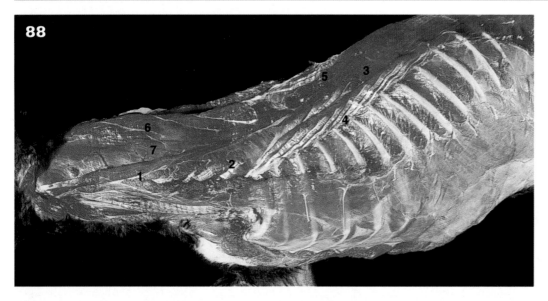

88

88   Lateral aspect of the deep epaxial muscles of the neck and thoracic region of a dog. The splenius cervicis and dorsal serratus cranialis muscles have been removed.

1 M. longissimus capitis	5 M. spinalis and M. semispinalis
2 M. longissimus cervicis	thoracis
3 Mm. longissimus thoracis and	6 M. semispinalis capitis (biventer)
lumborum	7 M. semispinalis capitis
4 M. iliocostalis thoracis	(complexus)

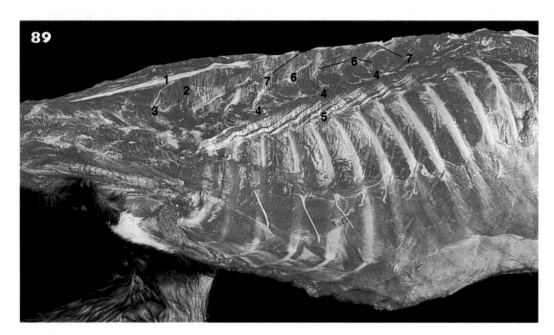

89

89   Lateral aspect of the deeper layer of the epaxial muscles of the neck and thorax of a dog. The semispinalis capitis and thoracis muscles have been removed to expose the ligamentum nuchae.

1 Ligamentum nuchae	5 M. iliocostalis thoradis
2 M. spinalis cervicis	6 Mm. interspinales
3 M. multifidus cervicis	7 Supraspinous ligament
4 M. multifidus thoracis	

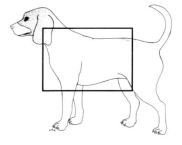

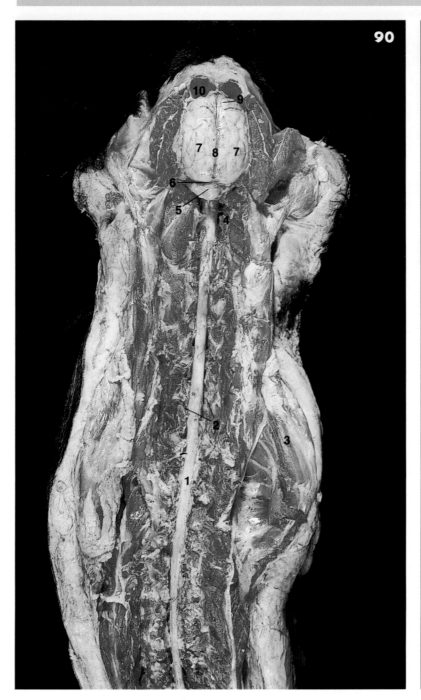

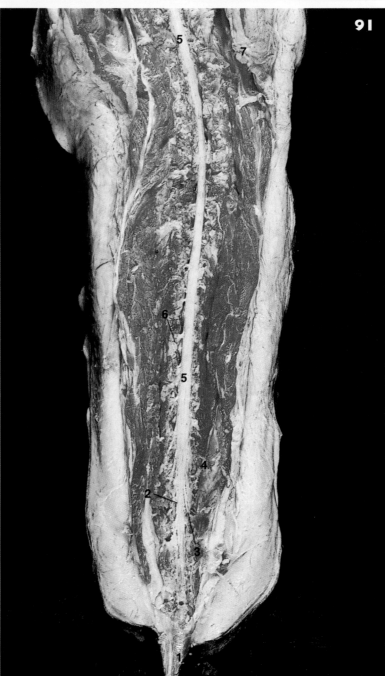

90   Dorsal aspect of the brain and spinal cord of a dog, to the level of the thoracolumbar junction. The dorsal epaxial muscles, the dorsal vertebral laminae, and the root of the cranium have been removed to reveal the meningeal layers covering the brain and spinal cord.

1	Dura mater covering spinal cord	7	Cerebral hemispheres
2	Vertebral canal	8	Sagittal sinus overlying
3	Pectoral limb		longitudinal fissure
4	First cervical vertebra (atlas)	9	Olfactory bulbs
5	Cerebellum	10	Frontal sinus
6	Transverse sinus overlying		
	transverse fissure		

91   Dorsal aspect of the spinal cord of a dog, from the level of the first thoracic vertebra. The dorsal epaxial muscles and the dorsal vertebral laminae have been removed to reveal the vertebral canal.

1	Tali	5	Dura mater covering spinal
2	Cauda equina		cord
3	Caudal spinal nerves	6	Spinal nerve
4	Sacrum	7	Pectoral limb

4 THORACIC LIMB

Beginning with the proximal structures and descending distally to the manus, the osteology and myology of the thoracic limb are displayed. The osteological details are revealed first, using bony specimens (both singly and in an articulated form) and radiographs, and the muscular attachments are then illustrated, followed by prepared dissections. Blood vessels and nerves are named as they occur in the dissections, and a contrast medium is used with radiography to explain the course of the vascular supply.

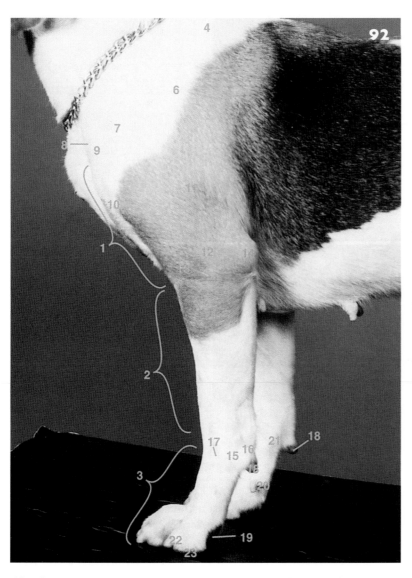

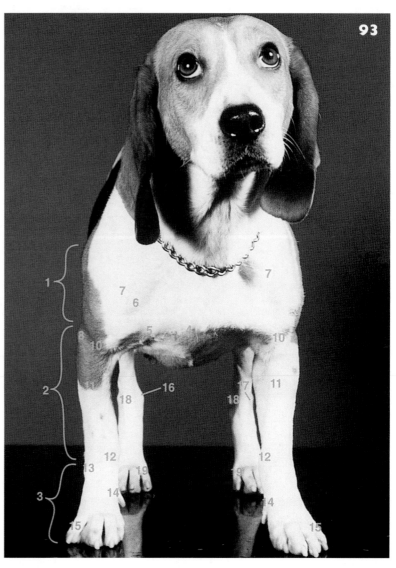

92 Lateral aspect of the left thoracic limb of a standing live dog, demonstrating palpable landmarks commonly used in clinical examination.

93 Cranial aspect of the thoracic limbs of a standing live dog, demonstrating palpable landmarks. The dorsal aspect of the pes of the pelvic limb is also displayed.

1 Brachium	13 Elbow joint (cubital joint)
2 Antebrachium	14 Olecranon process ⎫ of ulna
3 Manus	15 Styloid process ⎭
4 Cranial angle ⎫ of scapula	16 Accessory carpal bone
5 Caudal angle ⎭	17 Carpal joint
6 Spine	18 Carpal pad
7 Acromion	19 Metacarpal pad
8 Shoulder joint	20 First digit (dew claw)
9 Greater tubercle of humerus	21 Styloid process of radius
10 Deltoid tuberosity	22 Fifth digit
11 M. triceps brachii	23 Digital pad
12 Lateral epicondyle of humerus	

1 Brachium	11 Cephalic vein (in subcutaneous position)
2 Antebrachium	12 Styloid process of radius
3 Manus	13 Styloid process of ulna
4 Manubrium sterni	14 First digit
5 Pectoral muscle mass	15 Fifth digit
6 M. brachiocephalicus	16 Medial malleolus of tibia ⎫
7 Shoulder joint	17 Lateral malleolus of fibula ⎬ pelvic limb
8 Lateral epicondyle ⎫ of humerus	18 Tarsal joint (hock) ⎪
9 Medial epicondyle ⎭	19 Second digit ⎭
10 Elbow joint	

94

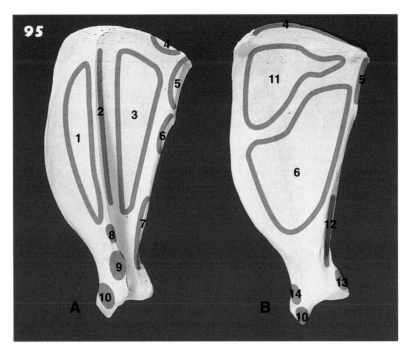

94 Lateral aspect of the left scapula (A) and medial aspect of the right scapula (B) of a dog.

1	Cranial angle
2	Dorsal border
3	Infraspinous fossa
4	Caudal angle
5	Caudal border
6	Spine
7	Acromion
8	Ventral angle
9	Supraglenoid tubercle
10	Scapular notch
11	Cranial border
12	Supraspinous fossa
13	Caudal border
14	Facies serrata
15	Subscapular fossa
16	Infraglenoid tubercle
17	Glenoid cavity
18	Supraglenoid tubercle
19	Coracoid process

95

95 Lateral (A) and medial (B) aspect of the scapula of a dog, showing areas of muscle attachment.

1	Supraspinatus	8	Omotransversarius
2	Trapezius and deltoideus	9	Deltoideus
3	Infraspinatus	10	Biceps brachii
4	Rhomboideus	11	Serratus ventralis
5	Teres major	12	Long head of triceps
6	Subecapularis	13	Teres minor
7	Terse minor and long head of triceps	14	Coracobrachialis

96 Lateral (A) and medial (B) aspect of the scapula of a dog, showing the centres of ossification.

1 Body
2 Supraglenoid tubercle

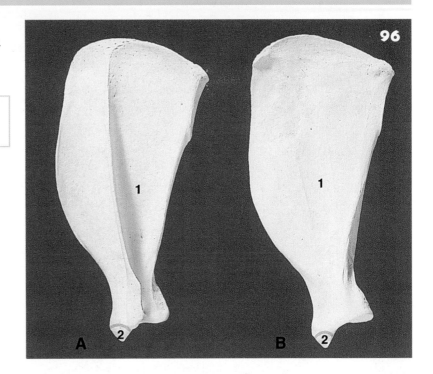

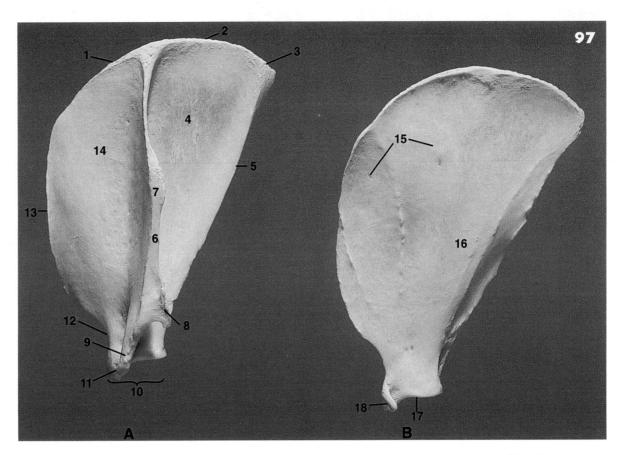

97 Lateral aspect of the left scapula (A) and medial aspect of the right scapula (B) of a cat.

1	Cranial angle	8	Suprahamate process }of acromion	14	Supraspinous fossa
2	Dorsal border			15	Facies serrata
3	Caudal angle	9	Hamate process	16	Subscapular fossa
4	Infraspinous fossa	10	Ventral angle	17	Glenoid cavity
5	Caudal border	11	Supraglenoid tubercle	18	Coracoid process
6	Spine	12	Scapular notch		
7	Tuberosity of spine	13	Cranial border		

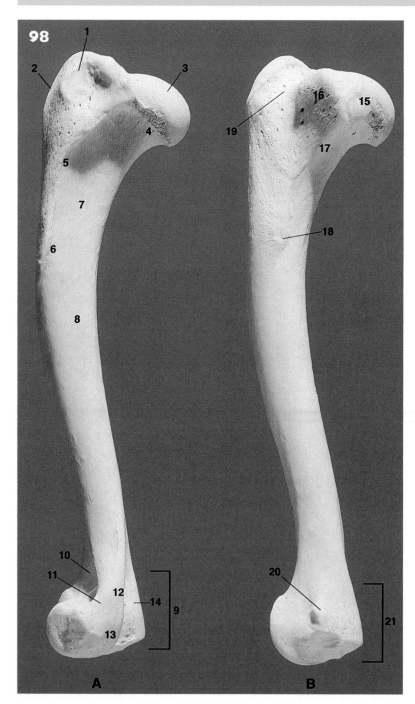

98   Lateral aspect of the left humerus (A) and medial aspect of the right humerus (B) of a dog.

1	Greater tubercle	11	Supratrochlear foramen
2	Crest of 1	12	Lateral epicondylar crest
3	Head	13	Lateral epicondyle
4	Neck	14	Olecranon fossa
5	Tricipital line (anconeal crest)	15	Head
6	Deltoid tuberosity	16	Lesser tubercle
7	Brachial groove (musculospiral groove)	17	Crest of 16
		18	Tuberosity for teres major
8	Body	19	Intertubercular groove
9	Condyle	20	Medial epicondyle
10	Radial fossa	21	Condyle

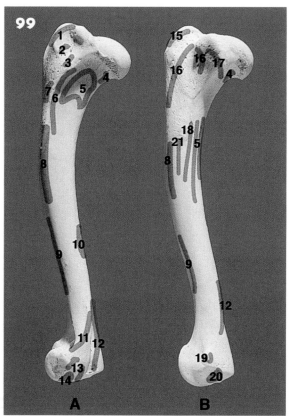

99   Lateral (A) and medial (B) aspect of the humerus of a dog, showing areas of muscle attachment.

1	Supraspinatus	13	Extensors of carpus and digits, and ulnaris lateralis
2	Infraspinatus		
3	Teres minor	14	Supinator
4	Accessory head of triceps	15	Supraspinatus
5	Brachialis	16	Pectoralis profundus
6	Lateral head of triceps	17	Subscapularis
7	Pectoralis superficialis	18	Coracobrachialis and medial head of triceps
8	Deltoideus		
9	Cleidobrachialis	19	Pronator teres
10	Brachioradialis	20	Flexors of carpus and digits
11	Extensor carpi radialis	21	Teres major and latissimus dorsi
12	Anconeus		

Clinical Note

8   Note that the body of the humerus is somewhat S-shaped in its contour and this presents problems with selecting an intramedullary pin to repair fractures of the shaft. An intramedullary pin is normally chosen so that it fills the diameter of the medullary cavity as fully as possible. However due to the S-shape of the humeral body or shaft a pin of a narrower calibre must be used in order that it can traverse down the curved medullary cavity. Fractures of the body tend to be distal in position due to the massive thickness of the bone proximally and the relative thinning distally, with the presence of the supratrochlear foramen and distal growth plate in young animals.

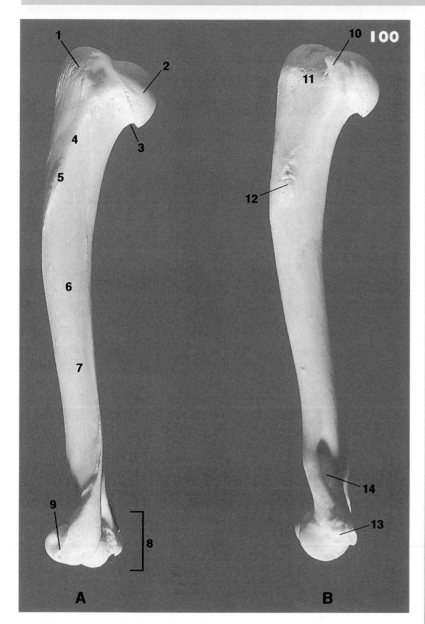

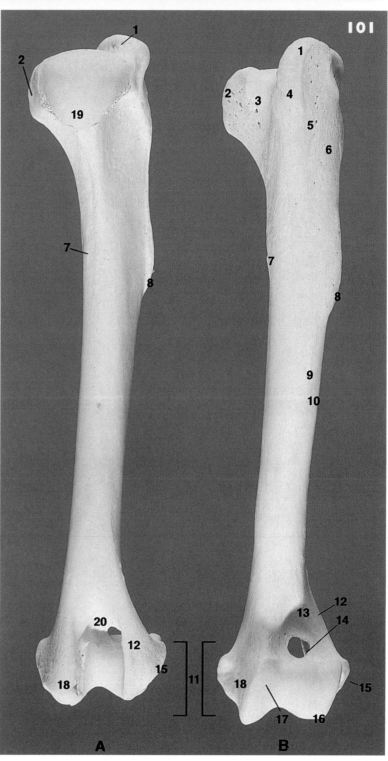

100 Lateral aspect of the left humerus (A) and medial aspect of the right humerus (B) of a cat.

1	Greater tubercle	8	Condyle
2	Head	9	Lateral epicondyle
3	Neck	10	Lesser tubercle
4	Tricipital line	11	Intertubercular groove
5	Deltoid tuberosity	12	Tuberosity for M. teres major
6	Body	13	Medial epicondyle
7	Brachial groove	14	Supracondylar foramen

101 Caudal aspect of the right humerus (A) and cranial aspect of the left humerus (B) of a dog.

1	Greater tubercle	11	Condyle
2	Lesser tubercle	12	Lateral epicondylar crest
3	Intertubercular groove	13	Radial fossa
4	Crest of greater tubercle	14	Supratrochlear foramen
5	Tuberosity for M. teres minor	15	Lateral epicondyle
6	Tricipital line	16	Capitulum
7	Tuberosity for M. teres major	17	Trochlea
8	Deltoid tuberosity	18	Medial epicondyle
9	Body	19	Head
10	Brachial groove	20	Olecranon fossa

Clinical Note

Fig. 100, 14 The presence of the supratrochlear foramen is a useful differential indicator when comparing the humerus of cat and dog. In life the brachial artery and median nerve pass through it so that a fracture at this point can have serious repercussions for the cat.

Fig. 101, 14 In some of the smaller short-leg breeds, e.g. Cairn terriers, a patent foramen may be missing. In life, no structures pass through the dog's foramen, which is bridged over by connective tissue.

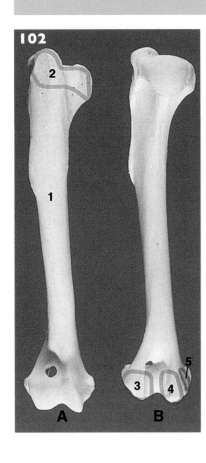

102   Cranial aspect of the right humerus (A) and caudal aspect of the left humerus (B) of a dog, showing the centres of ossification.

1	Body
2	Proximal
3	Lateral condyle
4	Medial condyle
5	Medial epicondyle

103   Cranial aspect of the left humerus (A) and caudal aspect of the right humerus (B) of a cat.

1	Greater tubercle
2	Lesser tubercle
3	Intertubercular groove
4	Crest of greater tubercle
5	Tricipital line
6	Tuberosity for M. teres major
7	Deltoid tuberosity
8	Body
9	Supracondylar foramen
10	Condyle
11	Radial fossa
12	Lateral epicondyle
13	Medial epicondyle
14	Trochlea
15	Capitulum
16	Head
17	Supracondylar foremen
18	Olecranon fossa

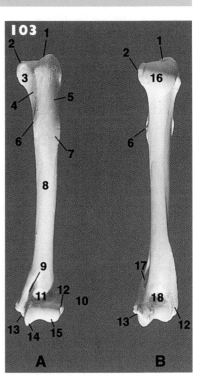

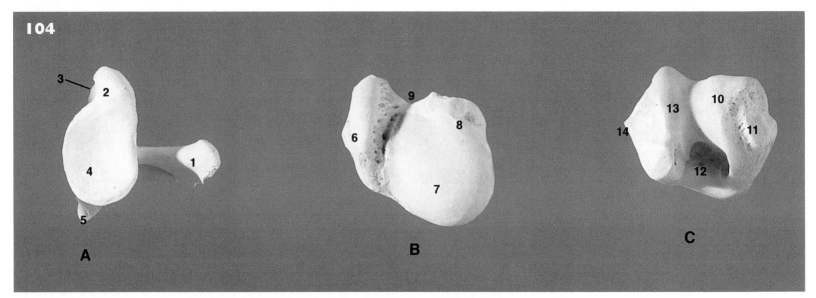

104   Distal extremity of the scapula (A), and proximal (B) and distal (C) extremities of the humerus of a dog.

1	Acromion process	8	Lesser tubercle
2	Supraglenoid tubercle	9	Intertubercular groove
3	Coracoid process	10	Capitulum
4	Glenoid cavity	11	Lateral eipicondyle
5	Infraglenoid tubercle	12	Olecranon fossa
6	Greater tubercle	13	Trochlea
7	Head	14	Medial epicondyle

Clinical Note
6 Note the groove immediately medial to the greater tubercle with its characteristic foraminae. It is through this groove that an intramedullary pin can be introduced and driven distally to effect immobilisation of a fracture of the body of the humerus.

105 Cranial aspect of the left shoulder joint (A) and caudal aspect of the right shoulder joint (B) of a dog.

1	Body of scapula	9	Intertubercular groove
2	Scapular spine	10	Tricipital line
3	Acromion	11	Body of humerus
4	Scapular notch	12	Neck of scapula
5	Supraglenoid tubercle	13	Infraglenoid tubercle
6	Coracoid process	14	Border of glenoid cavity
7	Greater tubercle	15	Head
8	Lesser tubercle		

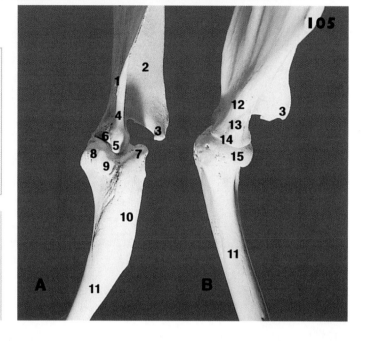

Clinical Note

3 & 7 Note the relative positions of these two palpable bony structures. They are used as palpable landmarks when assessing the correct position of the shoulder joint. In cases of dislocation of that joint there would be disparity in the relative approximation of these structures.

106 Lateral radiograph of the shoulder region. The cranially advanced limb is the lower limb in lateral recumbency. To enhance outline, the shoulder joint has been positioned so that its image is superimposed on that of the trachea.

1	Seventh cervical vertebra
2	First thoracic vertebra
3	First rib
4	Body of scapula
5	Scapular spine
6	Supraspinatous fossa
7	Infraspinatous fossa
8	Acramion process
9	Trachea
10	Supraglenoid tubercle
11	Infraglenoid tubercle
12	Glenoid cavity
13	Shoulder joint
14	Head of humerus
15	Greater tubercle
16	Body of humerus
17	Deltoid tuberosity
18	Elbow joint
19	Olecranon
20	Sternum
21	Heart
22	Bifurcation of 9
23	Oesophagus (gas filled)

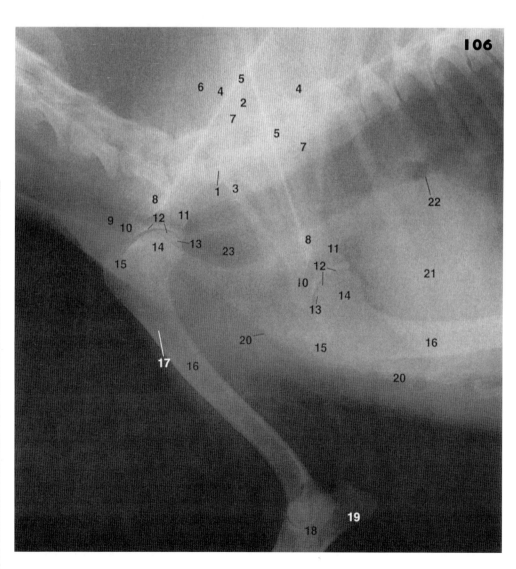

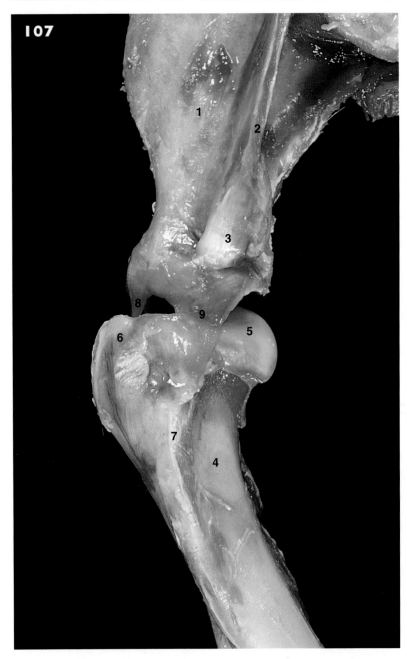

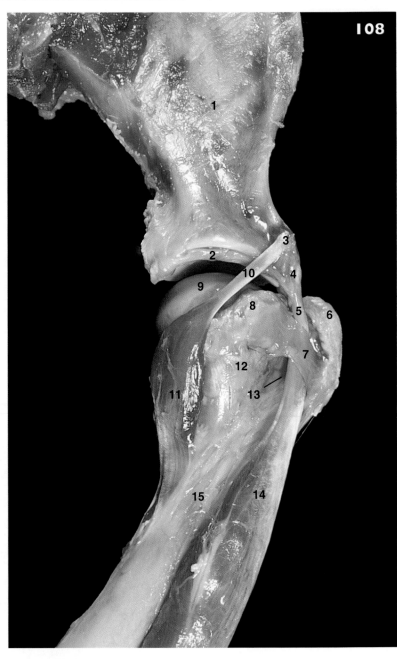

107   Lateral aspect of the left shoulder joint of a dog. The surrounding musculature has been dissected away to reveal the ligaments of the joint. The tendon of origin of the M. biceps brachii remains *in situ*.

1 Scapula	6 Greater tubercle
2 Spine of the scapula	7 Tricipital line
3 Acromion	8 Tendon of M. biceps brachii
4 Humerus	9 Lateral glenohumeral ligament
5 Head of humerus	

108   Medial aspect of the left shoulder joint of a dog. The surrounding musculature has been dissected away to reveal the ligaments of the joint. The tendon of origin of the M. biceps brachii remains *in situ*.

1 Scapula	9 Head of humerus
2 Glenoid cavity	10 Tendon of M. coracobrachialis
3 Coracoid process	11 M. coracobrachialis
4 Supraglenoid tubercle	12 Cut end of medial
5 Tendon of M. biceps brachii in	glenohumeral ligament
the intertubercular groove	13 Intertubercular groove
6 Greater tubercle	14 M. biceps brachii
7 Transverse humeral ligament	15 Humerus
8 Lesser tubercle	

109   Cranial aspect of the left shoulder joint of a dog. The surrounding musculature has been dissected away to reveal the ligaments of the joint. The tendon of origin of the M. biceps brachii remains *in situ*.

1 Scapula	8 Tendon of M. biceps brachii
2 Spine of scapula	9 Transverse humeral ligament
3 Acromion	10 Lesser tubercle
4 Glenoid cavity	11 Greater tubercle
5 Coracoid process	12 Humerus
6 Tendon of M. coracobrachialis	13 M. biceps brachii
7 Supraglenoid tubercle	14 M. coracobrachialis

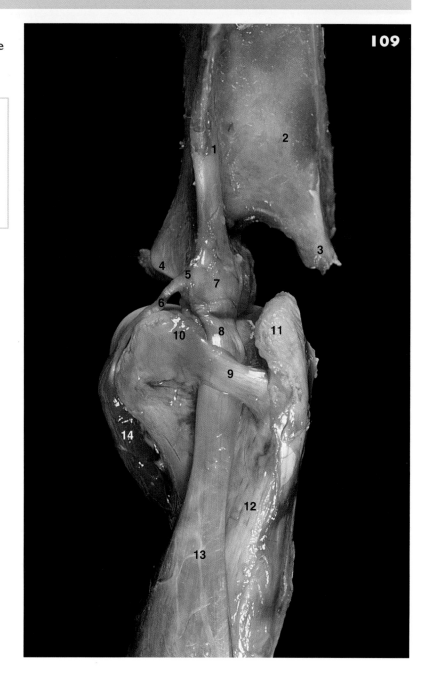

110

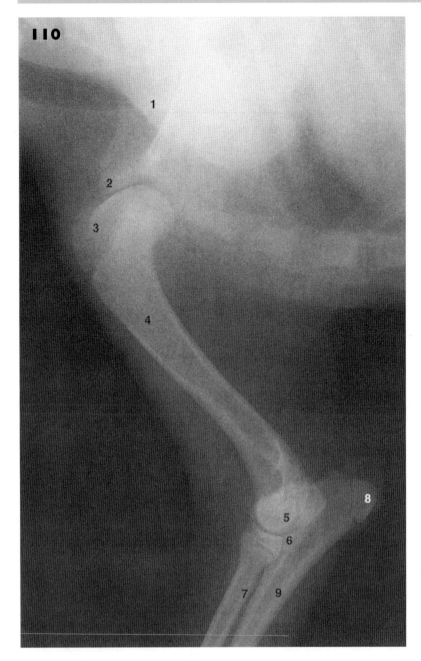

111

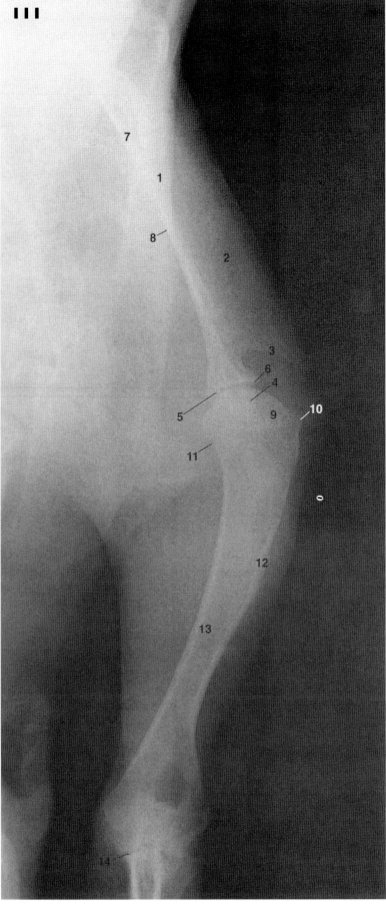

110   Mediolateral radiograph of the shoulder region of a puppy, showing the centres of ossification.

1   Body of scapula
2   Supraglenoid tubercle
3   Proximal humeral epiphysis
4   Body of humerus
5   Distal humeral epiphysis (combined)
6   Proximal radial epiphysis
7   Body of radius
8   Proximal ulnar epiphysis (precursor of olecranon)
9   Body of ulna

111   Caudocranial radiograph of the shoulder joint of a dog.

1   Body \
2   Spine / of scapula
3   Acromion
4   Supraglenoid tubercle with coracoid process
5   Glenoid cavity
6   Shoulder joint
7   Facies serrata
8   Subscapular fossa
9   Head of humerus
10 Greater tubercle
11 Lesser tubercle
12 Deltoid tuberosity
13 Body of humerus
14 Elbow joint (cubital joint)

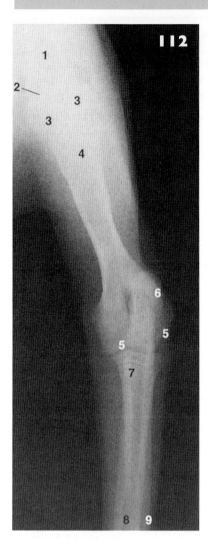

112

112   Craniocaudal radiograph of the shoulder and brachium of a puppy, showing the centres of ossification.

1   Body of scapula
2   Supraglenoid tubercle
3   Proximal humeral epiphysis
4   Body of humerus
5   Distal humeral epiphysis (combined)
6   Proximal ulnar epiphysis (precursor of olecranon)
7   Proximal radial epiphysis
8   Body of radius
9   Body of ulna

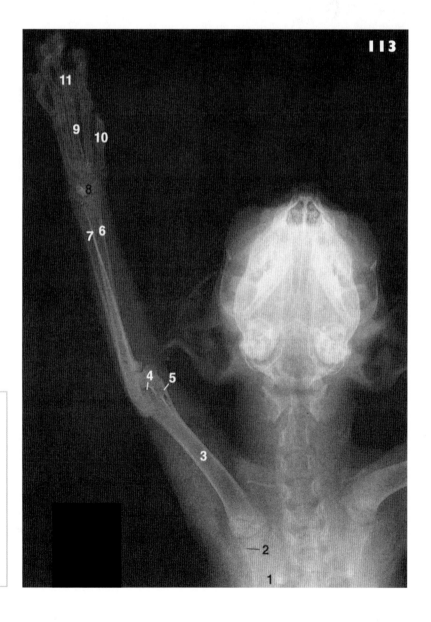

113

113   Craniocaudal radiograph of the thoracic limb of a kitten, showing the supracondylar foramen.

1   Scapula
2   Suprahamate process
3   Humerus
4   Supratrochlear fossa
5   Supracondylar foramen
6   Radius
7   Ulna
8   Carpus
9   Metacarpals
10   First digit
11   Second to fifth digits

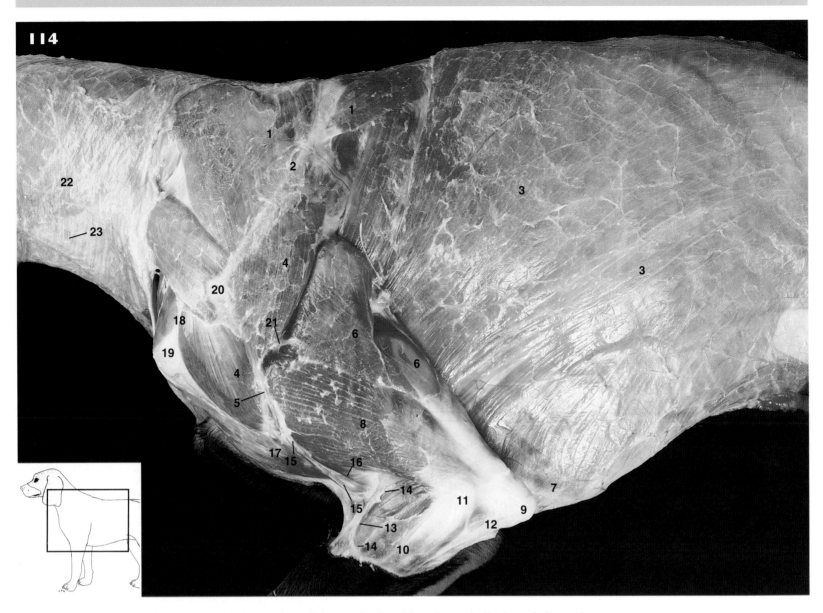

114   Lateral aspect of the superficial muscles of the neck, shoulder, thoracic limb and thoracic wall of a dog.

1 M. trapezius	9 Olecranon	17 M. cleidobrachialis
2 Scapular spine	10 Extensor group	18 M. supraspinatus
3 M. cutaneus trunci	11 Lateral epicondyle of humerus	19 Greater tubercle of humerus
4 M. deltoideus	12 M. anconeus	20 Acromion process
5 Axillobrachial vein	13 Superficial brachial artery	21 Cranial lateral cutaneous
6 M. triceps brachii (long head)	14 Radial nerve (superficial lateral	nerve (axillary)
7 M. pectoralis profundus (deep	and medial branches)	22 M. sphincter colli
to M. cutaneus trunci)	15 Cephalic vein	23 External jugular vein
8 M. triceps brachii (lateral head)	16 Median cubital vein	

Clinical Note

17   The sites for surgical incisions to carry out open reduction of fractures of the humeral body by intramedullary pinning are three in number. A proximal fracture is approached by separating the caudal edge of the M. cleidobrachialis from the cranial edge of the M. triceps (lateral head, 8). A mid-shaft fracture is approached by dividing the caudal edge of the M. cleidobrachialis from the cranial edge of the M. brachialis which is at the level marked 16. A distal fracture is approached by dividing between the caudal edge of the M. brachialis Tand the cranial ledge of the M. triceps at the level marked 14. Note the vulnerability of the radial nerve (14) to trauma at this point.

115   Medial aspect of the shoulder and brachium of the detached left thoracic limb of a dog. The extrinsic muscles have been sectioned.

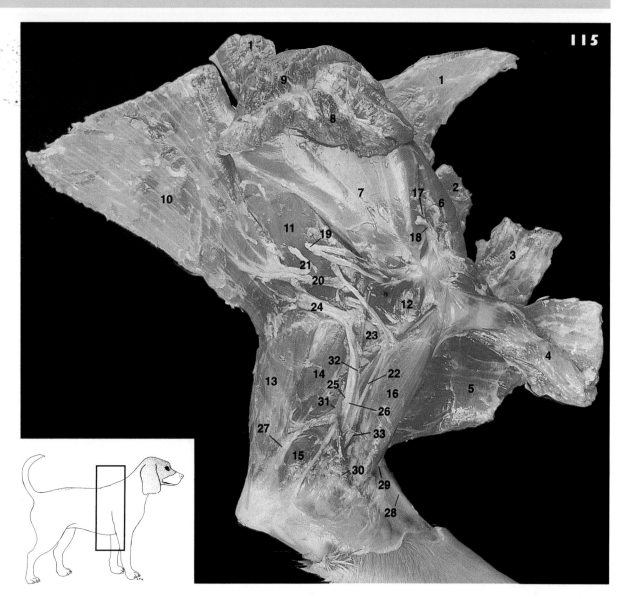

115

1	M. trapezius	12	M. coracobrachialis	23	Radial nerve
2	M. omotransversarius	13	M. tensor fasciae antebrachii	24	Median and ulnar nerve
3	M. cleidobrachialis with nerve	14	M. triceps brachii (long head)	25	Ulnar nerve
4	M. pectoralis profundus	15	M. triceps brachii (medial head)	26	Median nerve
5	M. pectorales superficiales	16	M. biceps brachii	27	Caudal cutaneous antebrachial nerve
6	M. supraspinatus	17	Subscapular nerve	28	Cephalic vein
7	M. subscapularis	18	Suprascapular nerve	29	Median cubital vein
8	M. serratus ventralis (cut edge)	19	Axillary nerve	30	Median vein
9	M. rhomboideus (cut edge)	20	Lateral thoracic nerve	31	Brachial vein
10	M. latissimus dorsi	21	Thoracodorsal nerve	32	Brachial artery
11	M. teres major	22	Musculocutaneous nerve	33	Bicipital artery

Clinical Note

17–27   These peripheral nerves all come from the brachial plexus which lies in the region of the axilla. The brachial plexus is supplied by the ventral branches of spinal nerves C5, 6, 7, 8 & T1. Severe trauma of the brachial plexus would result in motor dysfunction of all of the muscles shown here except the Mm. trapezius (1), omotransversarius (2) and rhomboideus (9), which receive motor nerve supply from dorsal branches of spinal nerves or the spinal accessory nerve (cranial nerve XI). In complete brachial plexus paralysis there would be a loss of sensation to stimulation to the skin over the lateral shoulder region, continuing distally and involving the whole limb surface distal to the elbow. This is a differential diagnosis point when testing between radial nerve and brachial plexus paralysis. In the former condition there would only be loss of sensation over the cranial antebrachium and dorsum of the manus.

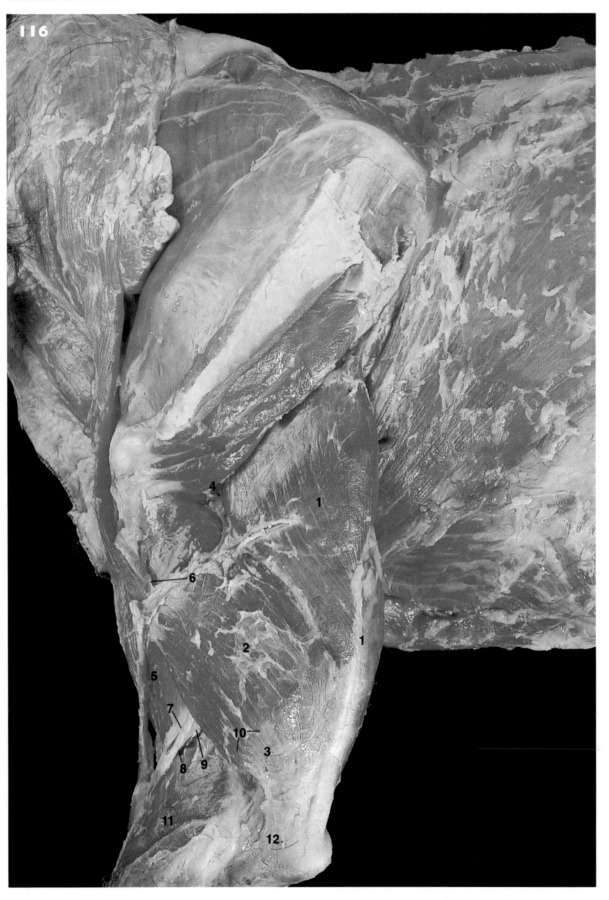

116

116   Lateral aspect of the deep muscles of left shoulder and brachium of a dog. The trapezius and deltoideus muscles have been resected.

1   M. triceps brachii (long head)
2   M. triceps brachii (lateral head)
3   M. triceps brachii (medial head)
4   M. teres minor
5   M. branchialis
6   Radial nerve
7   Medial branch ⎫ of superficial
8   Lateral branch ⎭ ramus
9   Deep ramus
10 Muscular branches to triceps
11 M. extensor carpi radialis
12 M. anconeus

Clinical Note
6   The radial nerve at this level is not so vulnerable to trauma but paralysis from damage here would result in loss of motor supply to the extensors of the elbow, carpus and digits producing an animal with severe dysfunction, unable to stabilise its elbow joint and lower limb. There would be loss of conscious sensation over the cranial antebrachium and dorsum of the manus.

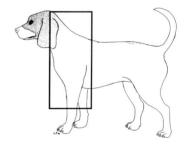

117 Lateral aspect of the deep muscles of the shoulder and brachium of the left thoracic limb of a dog. The omotransversarius, trapezius and deltoideus muscles, together with the lateral head of the triceps brachii, have been resected.

1 M. rhomboideus
2 M. latissimus dorsi
3 M. deltoideus (cut edge)
4 M. infraspinatus
5 M. teres minor
6 M. pectoralis profundus
7 M. triceps brachii (long head)
8 M. triceps brachii (accessory head)
9 M. extensor carpi radialis
10 M. anconeus
11 Radial nerve
12 M. brachialis
13 Cephalic vein
14 Axillobrachial vein
15 M. cleidobrachialis
16 Acromion process
17 Greater tubercle of humerus
18 M. supraspinatus
19 M. trapezius (cut edge)
20 M. omotransversarius (cut edge)
21 M. cleidocephalicus, pars cervicalis
22 Clavicular tendon

Clinical Note

5 The teres minor muscle crosses the lateral aspect of the shoulder joint. To gain surgical access from a lateral approach, the two heads of the deltoideus are divided to expose the teres minor, which is then rotated from its position or even sectioned to reveal the joint capsule.

11 The radial nerve is shown emerging from its spiralling passage through the brachial groove (musculospiral groove). In this position it is vulnerable to trauma at the time of fracture of the body of the humerus or during surgical repair of such a fracture. Testing for the functional status of the radial nerve can be carried out by stimulating the cranial and dorsal surfaces of the antebrachium and manus to exhibit a conscious reaction. A radial paralysis at this level would cause loss of motor function to the extensors of the carpus and digits but the motor supply to the M. triceps would still function and so the dog could still fix the elbow in extension. Thus the dog could maintain a near normal stance when immobile but on moving forward it would fail to extend the carpus and digits, producing a dragging of the limb with the dorsum of the manus in contact with the ground surface.

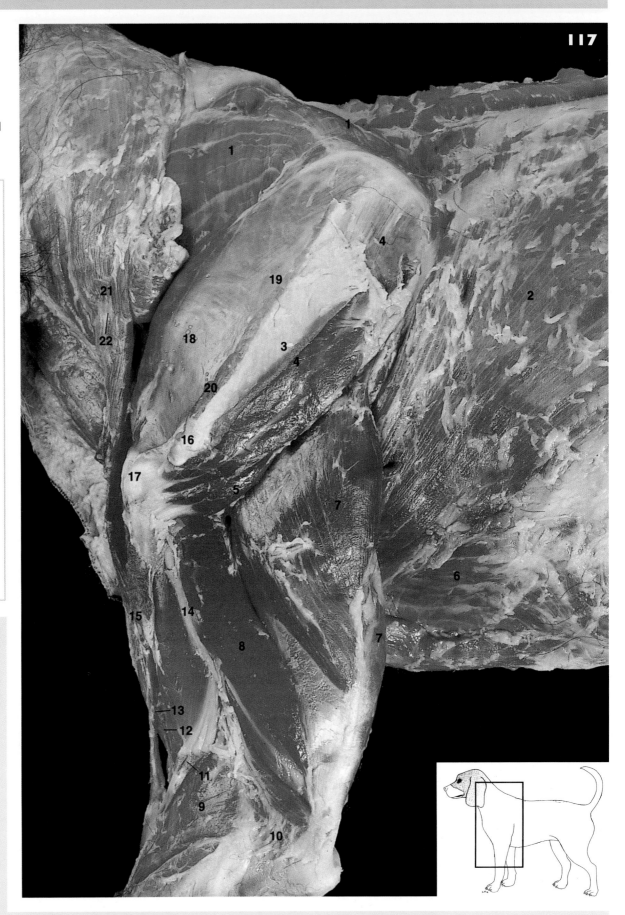

117

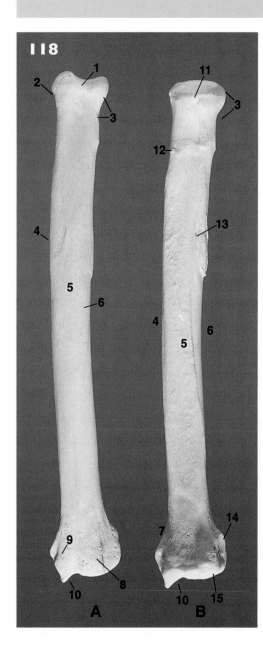

118 Cranial aspect of the left radius (A) and caudal aspect of the right radius (B) of a dog.

1 Fovea
2 Head
3 Neck
4 Medial border
5 Body
6 Lateral border
7 Groove for M. extensor digitalis communis
8 Groove for M. extensor carpi radialis
9 Groove for M. abductor pollicis longus
10 Styloid process
11 Articular circumference
12 Radial tuberosity
13 Nutrient foramen
14 Ulnar notch
15 Carpal articular surface

119 Cranial aspect of the left radius (A) and caudal aspect of the right radius (B) of a dog, showing the centres of ossification.

1 Body
2 Proximal
3 Distal

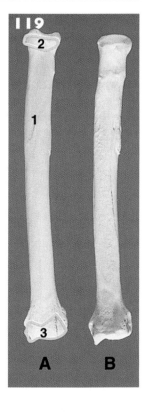

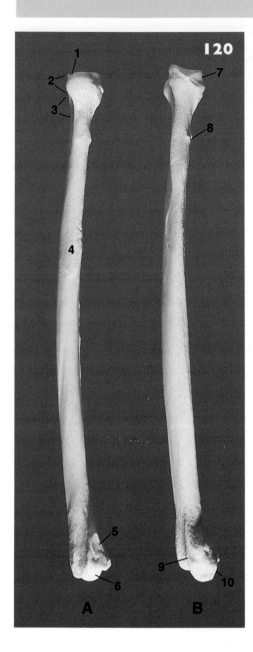

A   B

120

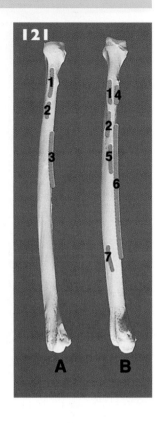

A   B

121

120   Lateral aspect of the left radius (A) and medial aspect of the right radius (B) of a dog.

1 Fovea
2 Head
3 Neck
4 Body
5 Ulnar notch
6 Carpal articular surface
7 Articular circumference
8 Radial tuberosity
9 Grooves for extensor muscles
10 Styloid process

121   Lateral (A) and medial (B) aspect of the radius of a dog, showing areas of muscle attachment.

1 Supinator
2 Pronator teres
3 Abductor pollicis longus
4 Biceps and brachialis
5 Flexor digitorum profundus
6 Pronator quadratus
7 Brachioradialis

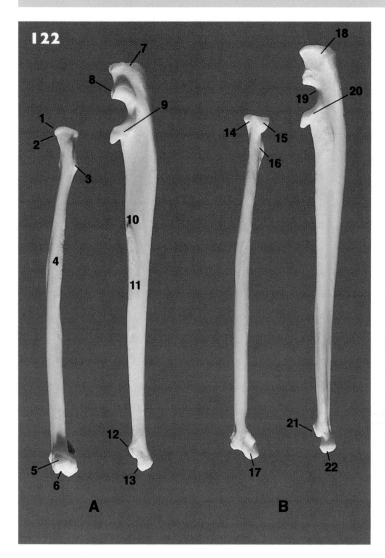

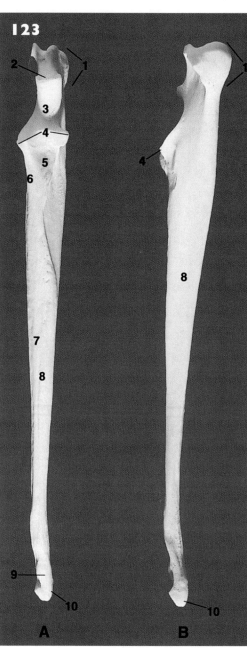

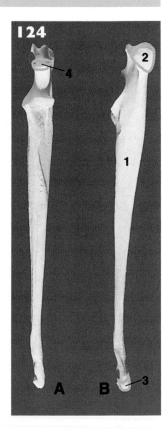

122   Lateral aspect of the left radius and ulna (A) and medial aspect of the right radius and ulna (B) of a cat.

1 Head ⎫ of radius	12 Ulnar notch
2 Neck ⎭	13 Styloid process of ulna
3 Radial tuberosity	14 Articular circumference
4 Body of radius	15 Articular fovea
5 Ulnar notch	16 Radial tuberosity
6 Carpal articular surface	17 Styloid process of radius
7 Olecranon of ulna	18 Olecranon
8 Anconeal process	19 Trochlear notch
9 Coronoid (lateral) process	20 Coronoid (medial) process
10 Interosseous border	21 Articular circumference
11 Body of ulna	22 Styloid process of ulna

124   Cranial aspect of the left ulna (A) and caudal aspect of the right ulna (B) of a dog, showing centres of ossification.

1 Body
2 Proximal
3 Distal
4 Anconeal (variable)

123   Cranial aspect of the left ulna (A) and caudal aspect of the right ulna (B) of a dog.

1 Olecranon
2 Anconeal process
3 Trochlear notch
4 Coronoid process
5 Radial notch
6 Ulnar tuberosity
7 Interosseous border
8 Body
9 Articular circumference
10 Styloid process

Clinical Note
4   It is around this articular surface that movement occurs during pronation and supination.

125 Lateral aspect of the left ulna (A) and medial aspect of the right ulna (B) of a dog.

1 Olecranon
2 Anconeal process
3 Trochlear notch
4 Coronoid process.
5 Radial notch
6 Body
7 Styloid process
8 Ulnar tuberosity
9 Interosseous border
10 Articular circumference

Clinical Note

2 The beak-like anconeal process in the standing position of extension of the elbow joint is located within the olecranon fossa of the humerus (see Figs 127, 130 & 132). This assists in stabilising the joint so that dislocation of this joint is uncommon and can only happen when the animal receives a blow with the joint in strong flexion or when trauma is accompanied by fracture of a humeral epicondyle.

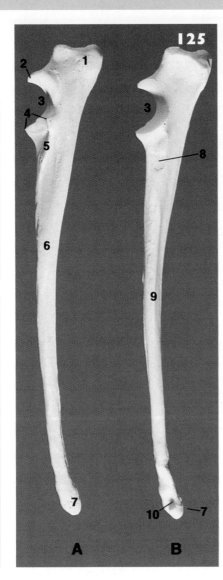

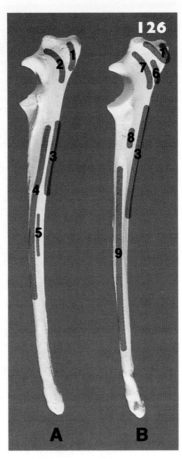

126 Lateral (A) and medial (B) aspect of the ulna, showing areas of muscle attachment.

1 Triceps
2 Anconeus
3 Flexor digitorum profundus
4 Abductor pollicis longus
5 Extensor pollicis longus
6 Tensor fasciae antebrachii
7 Flexor carpi ulnaris
8 Biceps branchii and branchialis
9 Pronator quadratus

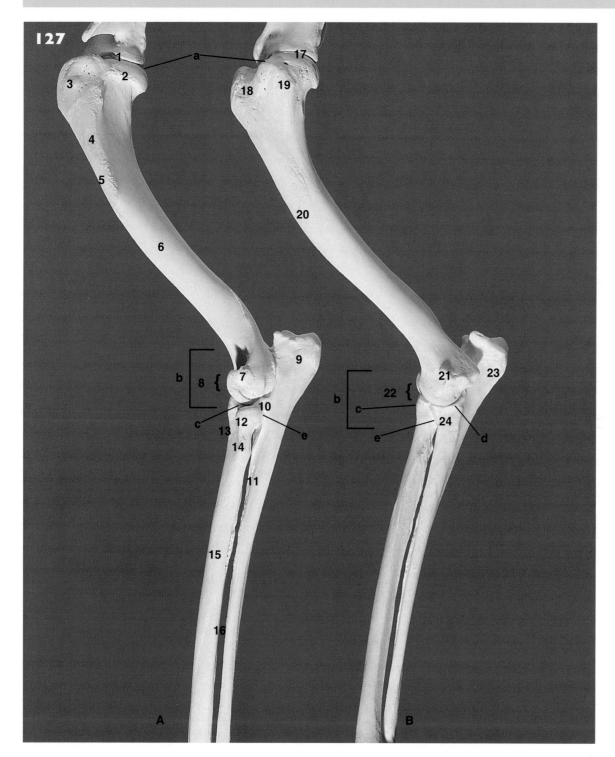

127   Lateral aspect of the left shoulder and elbow joint (A) and medial aspect of the right shoulder and elbow joint (B) of a dog.

a	Shoulder joint	6	Body of humerus	17	Shoulder joint space
b	Elbow joint (cubital joint)	7	Lateral epicondyle	18	Intertubercular groove
c	Humeroradial joint	8	Condyle	19	Lesser tubercle
d	Humero-ulnar joint	9	Olecranon	20	Body
e	Proximal radio-ulnar joint	10	Coronoid process	21	Medial epicondyle
		11	Body of ulna	22	Elbow joint space
		12	Fovea	23	Olecranon
1	Glenoid cavity	13	Head	24	Ulnar tuberosity
2	Head of humerus	14	Neck	of radius	
3	Greater tubercle	15	Body		
4	Tricipital line	16	Interosseous space		
5	Deltoid tuberosity				

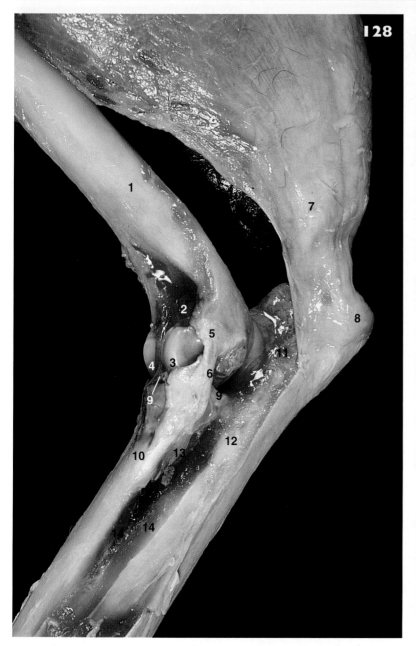

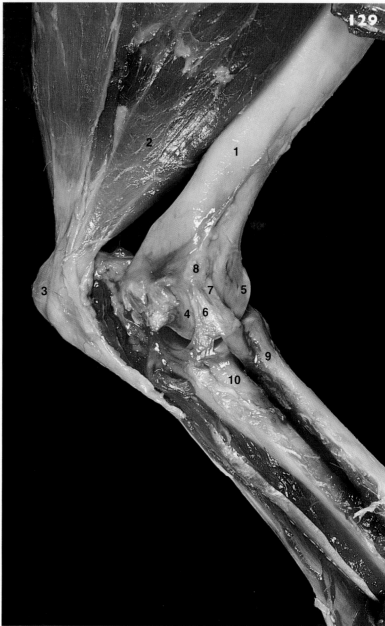

128   Lateral aspect of the left elbow joint of a dog. The M. triceps brachii has been left *in situ* after removal of the other surrounding musculature.

1	Humerus	8	Olecranon
2	Supratrochlear foramen	9	Annular ligament
3	Capitulum	10	Radius
4	Trochlea	11	Cut edge of M. anconeus
5	Lateral epicondyle	12	Ulna
6	Lateral collateral ligament	13	Interosseus membrane
7	M. triceps brachii	14	M. abductor pollicis longus

129   Medial aspect of the left elbow joint of a dog. The M. triceps brachii has been left *in situ* after removal of the other surrounding musculature.

1	Humerus	6	Medial collateral ligament
2	M. triceps brachii	7	Oblique ligament
3	Olecranon	8	Medial epicondyle
4	Trochlea	9	Radius
5	Capitulum	10	Ulna

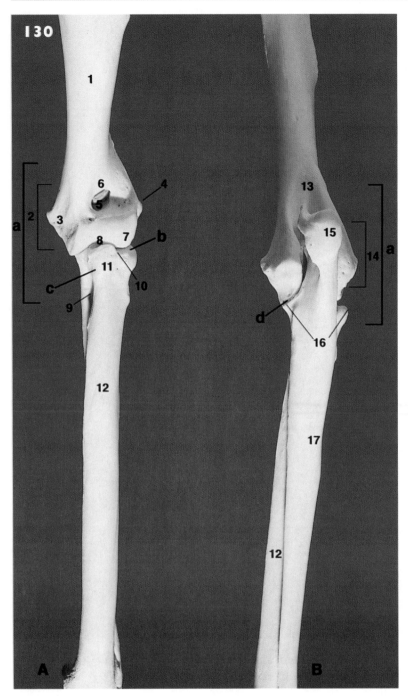

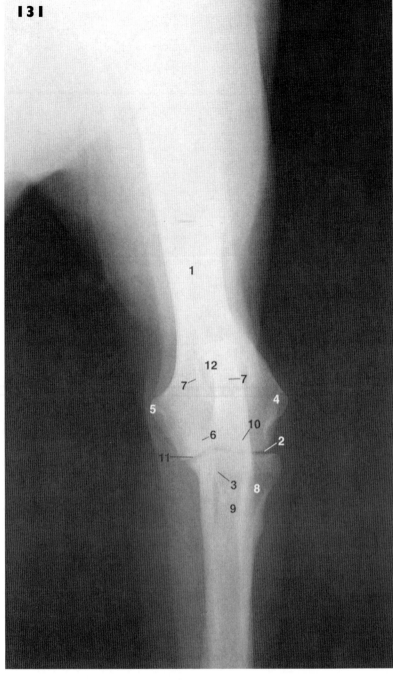

130   Cranial aspect of the left elbow joint (A) and caudal aspect of the right elbow joint (B) of a dog.

a	Elbow joint (cubital joint)	7	Capitulum
b	Humeroradial joint	8	Trochlea
c	Proximal radio-ulnar joint	9	Ulna
d	Humero-ulnar joint	10	Fovea
		11	Head ⎫ of radius
1	Body of humerus	12	Body ⎭
2	Condyle	13	Olecranon fossa
3	Medial epicondyle	14	Condyle
4	Lateral epicondyle	15	Olecranon
5	Supratrochlear foramen	16	Coronoid process
6	Radial fossa	17	Body of ulna

131   Craniocaudal radiograph of the elbow of a dog.

1	Body of humerus	7	Olecranon fossa
2	Elbow joint (cubital joint)	8	Radius
3	Proximal radio-ulnar joint	9	Ulna
4	Lateral epecondyle	10	Lateral coronoid process
5	Medial epicondyle	11	Medial coronoid process
6	Border of trochlea of humerus	12	Olecranon

132 Mediolateral radiograph of the antebrachium and carpus of a dog.

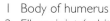

1 Body of humerus
2 Elbow joint (cubital joint)
3 Proximal radio-ulnar joint
4 Lateral part of capitulum
5 Medial part of trochlea of humerus
6 Lateral epicondyle
7 Lateral epicondylar crest
8 Medial epicondyle
9 Medial border of supratrochlear foramen
10 Radial tuberosity
11 Lateral coronoid process
12 Medial coronoid process
13 Anconeal process
14 Craniolateral tuberosity ⎫
15 Craniomedial tuberosity ⎬ of olecranon
    ⎭
16 Olecranon
17 Body of radius
18 Body of ulna
19 Interosseous space
20 Radial ⎫
21 Ulnar ⎪
22 Accessory ⎪
23 First ⎬ carpal bone
24 Second ⎪
25 Third ⎪
26 Fourth ⎭
27 Sesamoid bone in tendon of M. abductor pollicis longus
28 Distal radio-ulnar joint
29 Antebrachiocarpal joint
30 Middle carpal joint
31 Carpometacarpal joint
32 Styloid process of radius
33 Styloid process of ulna
34 First metacarpal bone
35 Second to fifth metacarpal bones
36 Carpal pad
37 Proximal sesamoid (palmar) ⎫
38 First phalanx ⎬ of first digit
39 Third phalanx ⎭
40 Proximal sesamoid (palmar)

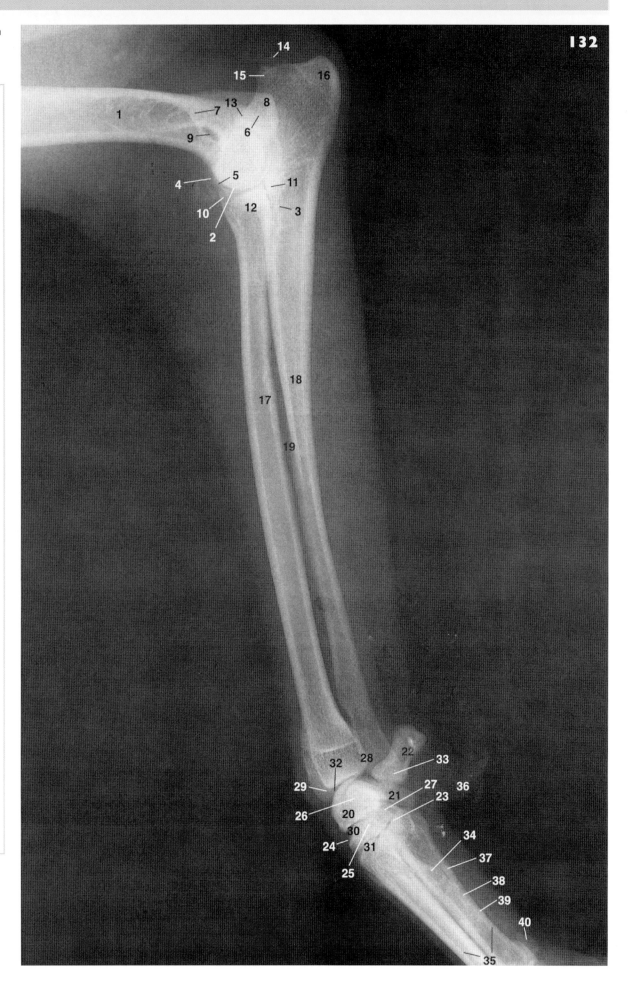

132

133

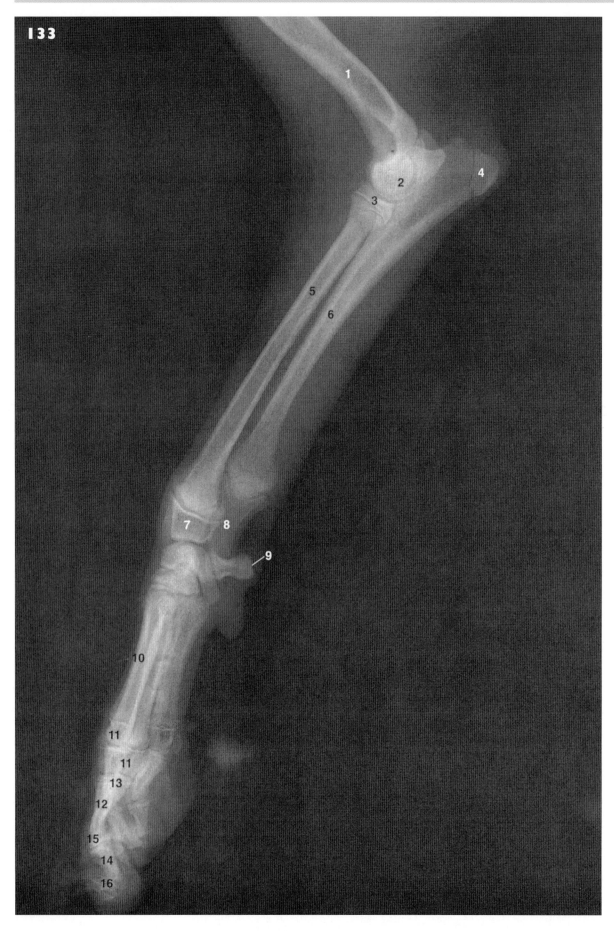

133   Mediolateral radiograph of the antebrachium, carpus and manus of a puppy, showing centres of ossification.

1   Body of humerus
2   Distal humeral epiphysis (combined)
3   Proximal radial epiphysis
4   Proximal ulnar epiphysis (precursor of olecranon)
5   Body of radius
6   Body of ulna
7   Distal radial epiphysis
8   Distal ulnar epiphysis
9   Free epiphysis of accessory carpal bone
10 Body of metacarpus
11 Distal metacarpal epiphysis
12 Body of first phalanx
13 First phalangeal proximal epiphysis
14 Body of second phalanx
15 Second phalangeal proximal epiphysis
16 Body of third phalanx

Clinical Note
4   The centre for the olecranon is normally the only centre of ossification at the proximal end of the ulna. It is vulnerable to distraction in the young dog due to the strong pull of the M. triceps during extension of the elbow joint. On occasions a separate centre can be found for the anconeal process (13 in Fig. 132) which, if it fails to unite with the diaphysis, can produce pathological changes within the joint. This condition has a breed predisposition, e.g. German Shepherd dogs.
9   Note that the accessory carpal bone has two centres of ossification. As the major flexors of the carpus attach here it is vulnerable to distraction.

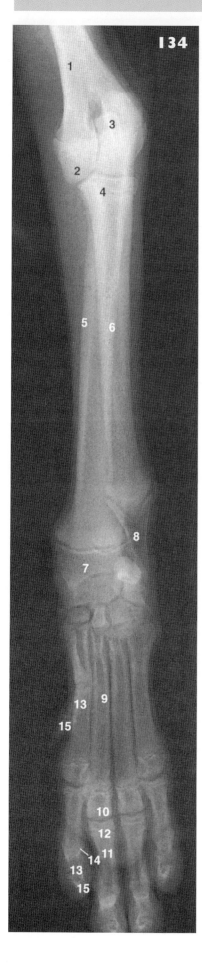

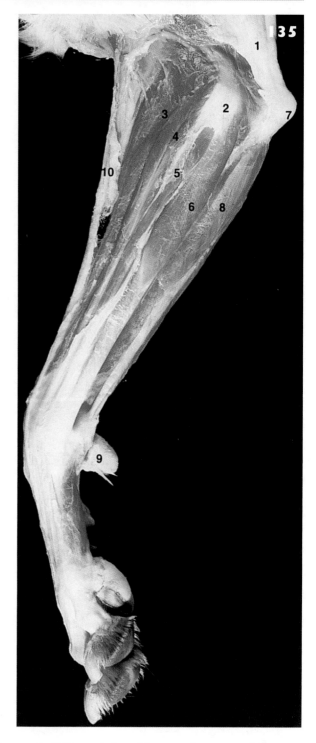

134   Dorsopalmar radiograph of the antebrachium, carpus and manus of a puppy, showing centres of ossification.

1 Body of humerus
2 Distal humeral epiphysis (combined)
3 Proximal ulnar epiphysis (precursor of olecranon)
4 Proximal radial epiphysis
5 Body of radius
6 Body of ulna
7 Distal radial epiphysis
8 Distal ulnar epiphysis
9 Body of metacarpus
10 Distal metacarpal epiphysis
11 Body of first phalanx
12 First phalangeal proximal epiphysis
13 Body of second phalanx
14 Second phalangeal proximal epiphysis
15 Body of third phalanx

135   Lateral aspect of the antebrachium and manus of the left thoracic limb of a dog.

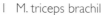

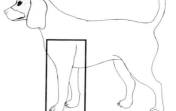

1 M. triceps brachil	6 M. extensor carpi ulnaris (M. ulnaris lateralis)
2 Lateral epicondyle of humerus	7 Olecranon
3 M. extensor carpi radialis	8 M. flexor carpi ulnaris (ulnar head)
4 M. extensor digitorum communis	9 Carpal pad
5 M. extensor digitorum lateralis	10 Cephalic vein

Clinical Note
2 Note that all of the extensors of the carpus and digits have an origin from the lateral epicondyle. This is a useful *aide-mémoire* when trying to allocate names and function to the muscles of the region.

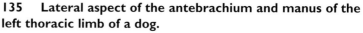

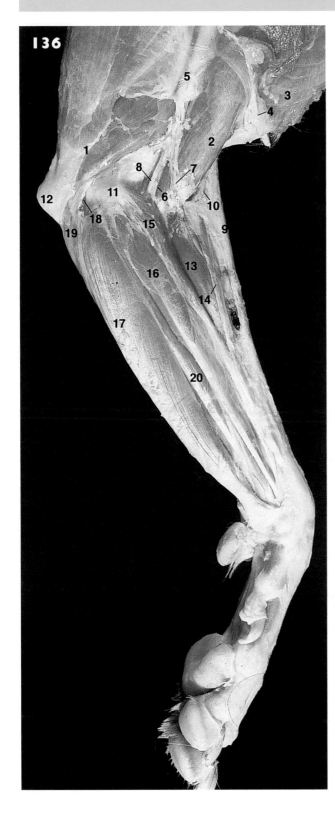

136   Medial aspect of the antebrachium and manus of the left thoracic limb of a dog. The limb has been removed from its attachment to the trunk.

1   M. triceps brachii
2   M. biceps brachii
3   Mm. pectorales superiores
4   Pectoral nerve
5   Brachial vein
6   Brachial artery
7   Superficial radial artery
8   Median nerve
9   Cephalic vein
10   Medial branch of superficial ramus of radial nerve
11   Medial epicondyle of humerus
12   Olecranon
13   M. extensor carpi radialis
14   M. brachioradialis
15   M. pronator teres
16   M. flexor carpi radialis
17   M. flexor digitorum superficialis
18   Ulnar nerve
19   M. flexor carpi ulnaris (ulnar head)
20   M. flexor digitorum profundus (humeral head)

Clinical Note
11   Note that all of the flexors of the carpus and digits have an origin from the medial epicondyle. This is a useful *aide-mémoire* when trying to allocate names and function to the muscles of the region.

137   Cranial aspect of the antebrachium and dorsal aspect of the manus of the left thoracic limb of a dog.

1   M. extensor carpi radialis
2   M. brachioradialis
3   Cephalic vein
4   Medial and lateral branches of superficial ramus of radial nerve
5   M. extensor digitorum communis
6   M. extensor digitorum lateralis
7   M. abductor pollicis longus
8   Tendon of M. extensor carpi lateralis (M. ulnar lateralis)
9   Tendon of 6
10   Tendon of 5
11   Site of dorsal sesamoid
12   Extensor tendon
13   Accessory cephalic vein
14   Dorsal metacarpal veins
15   Dorsal common digital arteries, veins and nerves

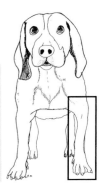

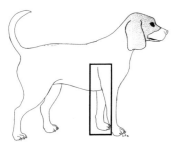

Clinical Note
3   This is the position at which venepuncture is frequently performed in the dog and cat. Note the close proximity of the medial and lateral branches of the superficial ramus of the radial nerve (4). The parallel course of the nerves to the vein can cause problems if there is leakage of potentially irritant pharmaceutical preparations perivenously. The animals will often self-mutilate the skin around the injection site, producing deep ulceration.

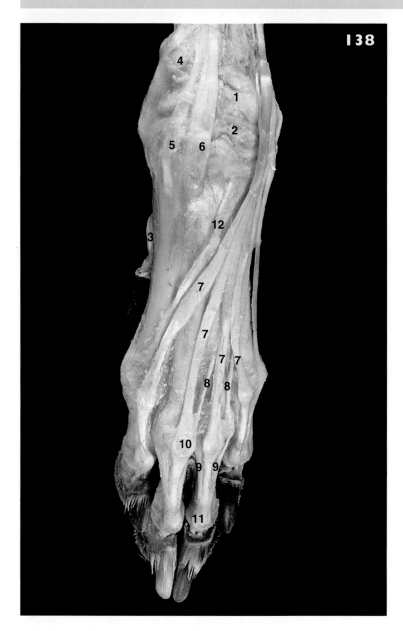

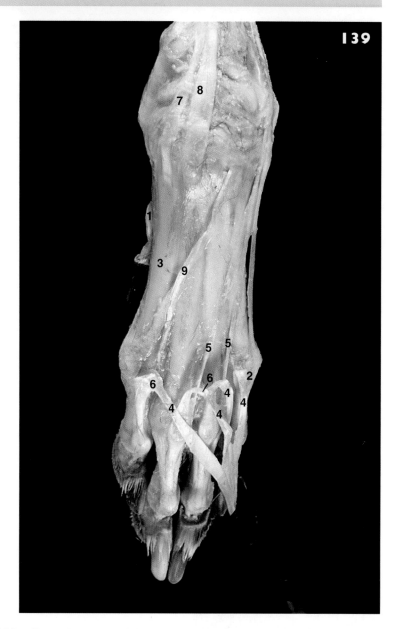

138   Dorsal aspect of the carpus and manus of the left thoracic limb of a dog. The tendons of the extensor muscles of the carpus and digits have been exposed by removal of the M. abductor pollicis longus.

139   Dorsal aspect of the carpus and manus of the left thoracic limb of a dog. The tendon of the common digital extensor muscle has been cut proximally and reflected distally.

1	Proximal row of carpal bones
2	Distal row of carpal bones
3	First digit
4	Position of sesamoid in tendon of M. abductor pollicis longus
5	Tendon of M. extensor carpi radialis (longus)
6	Tendon of M. extensor carpi radialis (brevis)
7	Tendons of M. extensor digitorum communis
8	Tendons of M. extensor digitorum lateralis
9	Tendons of Mm. interossei as they travel from the palmar to the dorsal aspect to become confluent with 7
10	Position of dorsal sesamoid
11	Dorsal elastic ligament
12	Tendon of M. extensor pollicis longus and indicis proprius

1	First digit
2	Fifth digit
3	Second metacarpal bone
4	Tendons of M. extensor digitorum communis
5	Tendons of M. extensor digitorum lateralis
6	Position of dorsal sesamoid in tendon of 4
7	Tendon of M. extensor carpi radialis (longus)
8	Tendon of M. extensor carpi radialis (brevis)
9	Tendon of the M. extensor pollicis longus and indicis proprius

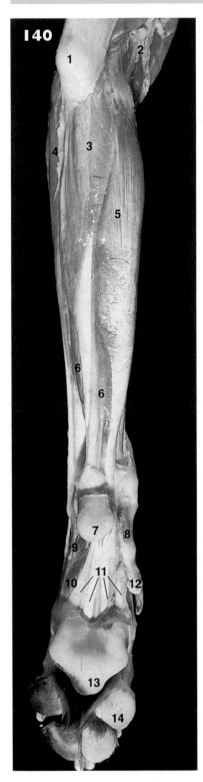

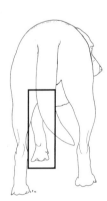

140   Caudal aspect of the antebrachium and palmar aspect of the manus of the left thoracic limb of a dog. The pads have been left intact.

1 Olecranon	7 Carpal pad
2 Median vessels	8 M. abductor pollicis brevis
3 M. flexor carpi ulnaris (ulnar head)	9 M. abductor digiti quinti
	10 M. flexor digiti quinti
4 M. extensor carpi ulnaris (M. ulnaris lateralis)	11 Tendons of 5
	12 First digit
5 M. flexor digitorum superficialis	13 Metacarpal pad
6 M. flexor carpi ulnaris (humeral head)	14 Digital pads

141   Dorsal aspect of the left carpus of a dog, in the articulated (A) and the separated (B) form.

1 Radial	⎫
2 Ulnar	⎪
3 Accessory	⎪
4 First	⎬ carpal bone
5 Second	⎪
6 Third	⎪
7 Fourth	⎭
8 Articular facet for radius	
9 Lateral process of 2	

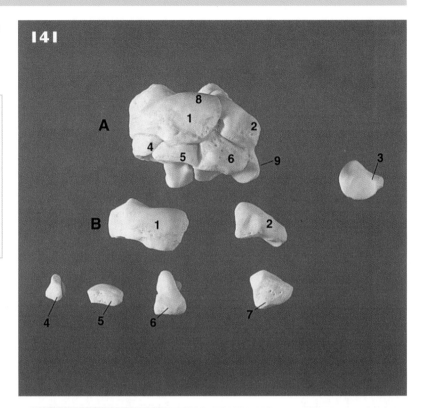

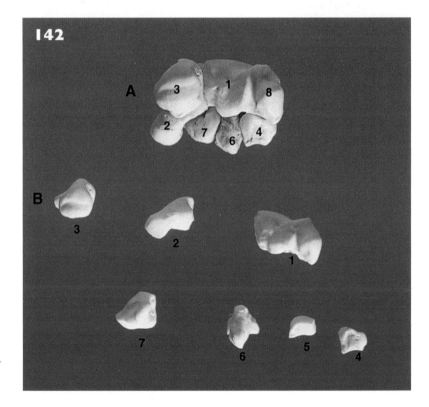

142   Palmar aspect of the left carpus of a dog in the articulated (A) and the separated (B) form.

1 Radial	⎫
2 Ulnar	⎪
3 Accessory	⎪
4 First	⎬ carpal bone
5 Second	⎪
6 Third	⎪
7 Fourth	⎭
8 Sulcus for tendon of M. flexor carpi radialis	

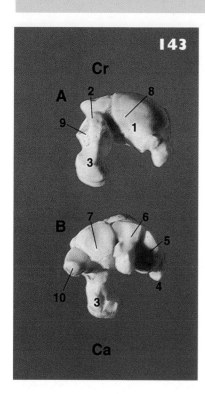

143 Proximal aspect of the left carpus (A) and distal aspect of the right carpus (B) of a dog, oriented cranially (Cr) and caudally (Ca).

1 Radial ⎫
2 Ulnar ⎪
3 Accessory ⎪
4 First ⎬ carpal bone
5 Second ⎪
6 Third ⎪
7 Fourth ⎭
8 Articular face for radius
9 Articular face for ulna
10 Palmar process of 2

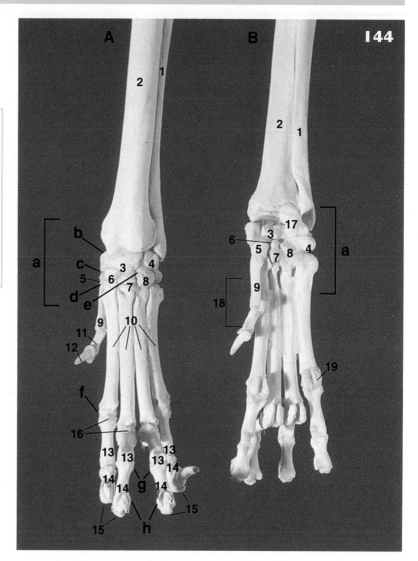

144 Dorsal aspect of the left carpus and manus (A), and palmar aspect of the right carpus and manus (B) of a dog.

a Carpal joints
b Antebrachiocarpal joint
c Middle carpal joint
d Carpometacarpal joints
e Intercarpal joints
f Metacarpophalangeal joints
g Proximal interphalangeal joint
h Distal interphalangeal joint

1 Body of ulna
2 Body of radius
3 Radial ⎫
4 Ulnar ⎪
5 First ⎪
6 Second ⎬ carpal bone
7 Third ⎪
8 Fourth ⎭

9 First metacarpal bone
10 Second to fifth metacarpal bones
11 Proximal phalanx ⎫ of first
12 Distal phalanx ⎭ digit
13 Proximal phalanges ⎫
  ⎪ of second
14 Middle phalanges ⎬ to fifth
  ⎪ digits
15 Distal phalanges ⎭
16 Dorsal sesamoids
17 Accessory carpal bone
18 First digit
19 Palmar sesamoids

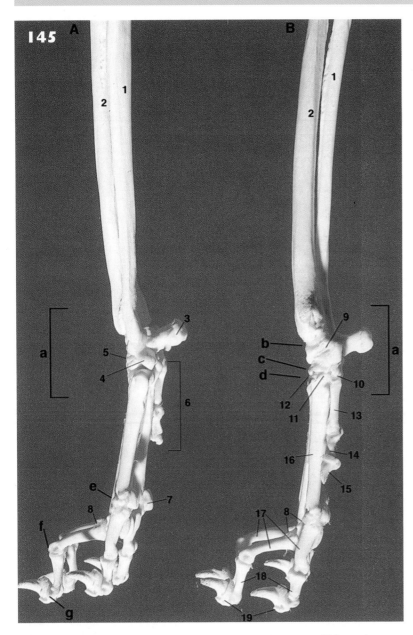

145   Lateral aspect of the left carpus and manus (A), and medial aspect of the right carpus and manus (B) of a dog.

a	Carpal joints	7	Palmar sesamoids
b	Antebrachiocarpal joint	8	Dorsal sesamoids
c	Middle carpal joint	9	Radial ⎫
d	Carpometacarpal joints	10	First ⎪
e	Metacarpophalangeal joint	11	Second ⎬ carpal bone
f	Proximal interphalangeal joint	12	Third ⎭
g	Distal interphalangeal joint	13	First metacarpal bone
		14	Proximal phalanx ⎫ of first
1	Body of ulna	15	Distal phalanx ⎭ digit
2	Body of radius	16	Second metacarpal bone
3	Accessory ⎫	17	Proximal phalanges ⎫ of second
4	Ulnar ⎬ carpal bone	18	Middle phalanges ⎬ to fifth
5	Fourth ⎭	19	Distal phalanges ⎭ digits
6	First digit		

146   Dorsopalmar radiograph of the carpus and manus of a dog.

1   Body of radius
2   Body of ulna
3   Styloid process of radius
4   Styloid process of ulna
5   Distal radio-ulnar joint
6   Antebrachiocarpal joint
7   Radial ⎫
8   Ulnar ⎪
9   Accessory ⎪
10   First ⎬ carpal bone
11   Second ⎪
12   Third ⎪
13   Fourth ⎭
14   Middle carpal joint
15   Carpometacarpal joint
16   Sesamoid in the tendon of
      M. abductor pollicis longus
17   First ⎫
18   Second ⎪
19   Third ⎬ metacarpal bone
20   Fourth ⎪
21   Fifth ⎭
22   Proximal sesamoids (palmar)
23   Dorsal sesamoid
24   Metacarpophalangeal joint
25   Proximal phalanx of first to
      fifth digits
26   Proximal interphalangeal joint
27   Middle phalanx of second to
      fifth digits
28   Distal interphalangeal joint
29   Distal phalanx of first to fifth
      digits
30   Ungual crest
31   Ungual process

Clinical Note

16   The tendon of insertion of the M. abductor pollicis longus has an intercalated sesamoid bone as the tendon passes from lateral to medial over the radial carpal bone. Care should be taken to identify this structure as a normal feature and not as a chip fracture.

23   Each tendon of insertion of the M. extensor digitorum communis passes over a dorsal sesamoid at the level of the metacarpophangeal joint (see Fig. 144, **16**). This should be recognised as a normal feature in canine radiographs of this region. A similar situation occurs in the cat but the sesamoid is commonly cartilaginous in nature.

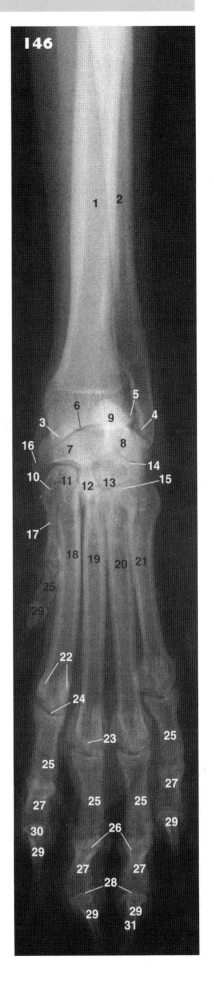

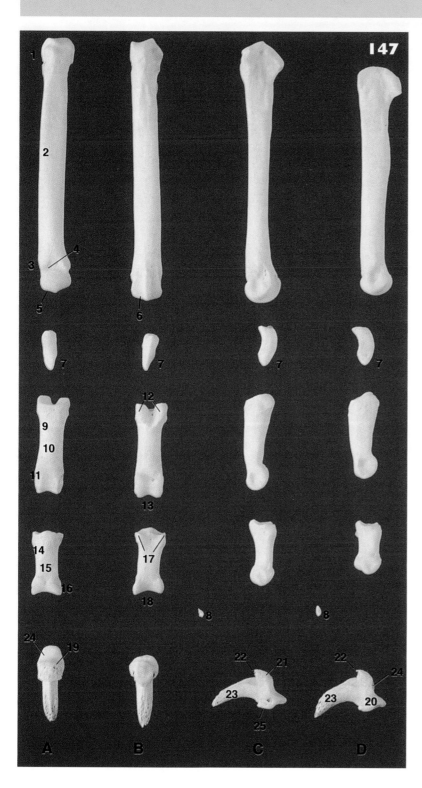

147

147   Dorsal (A), palmar (B), axial (C) and abaxial (D) aspects of the bones of a typical digit in the manus of a dog.

1 Base ⎫	17 Fovea with palmar tubercles
2 Body ⎬ of metacarpal	and sagittal ridge
3 Head ⎭	18 Trochlea
4 Sesamoid fossa	19 Base ⎫
5 Trochlea	20 Body ⎬ of distal phalanx
6 Sesamoid crest	21 Extensor tubercle
7 Proximal sesamoid	22 Ungual crest
8 Dorsal sesamoid	23 Ungual process
9 Base ⎫	24 Articular surface
10 Body ⎬ of proximal phalanx	25 Insertion of M. flexor
11 Head ⎭	digitorum profundus
12 Fovea with palmar tubercles	
13 Trochlea	
14 Base ⎫	
15 Body ⎬ of middle phalanx	
16 Head ⎭	

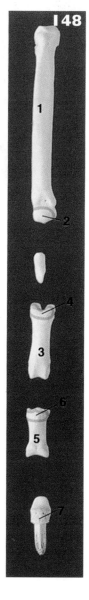

148

148   Dorsal aspect of a typical digit in the manus of a dog, showing centres of ossification.

1 Body of metacarpus
2 Distal metacarpus
3 Body of proximal phalanx
4 Proximal centre of proximal phalanx
5 Body of middle phalanx
6 Proximal centre of middle phalanx
7 Body of distal phalanx

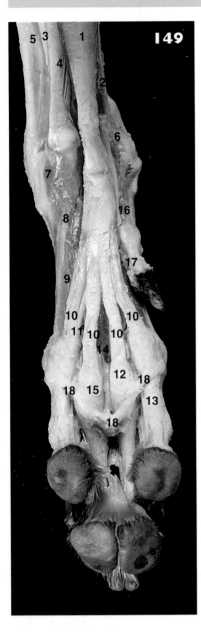

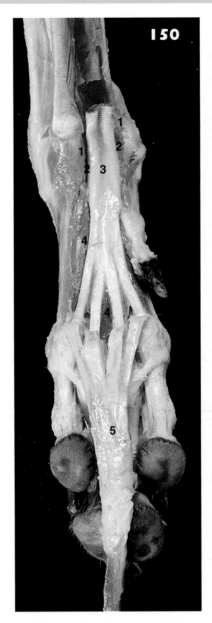

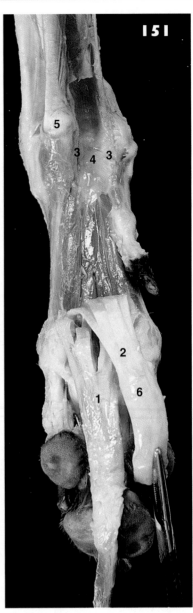

149 Palmar aspect of the manus of the left thoracic limb of a dog. The tendons of the superficial digital flexor have been dissected out as they course over the carpal region and into the manus. The carpal and metacarpal pads have been removed.

1 M. flexor digitorum superficialis
2 M. flexor carpi radialis
3 M. flexor carpi ulnaris (humeral head)
4 Tendon of M. flexor carpi ulnaris (ulnar head)
5 M. extensor carpi lateralis (M. ulnaris lateralis)
6 Carpal fascia (flexor retinaculum)
7 M. abductor digiti quinti
8 M. flexor digiti quinti
9 Fourth M. interosseus
10 Tendons of 1
11 One of the tendons of M. flexor digitorum profundus lying deep to 10
12 Palmar annular ligament (superficial transverse metacarpal ligament)
13 Proximal digital annular ligament
14 Mm. lumbricales
15 Position of proximal sesamoids
16 M. abductor pollicis brevis
17 Tendon of M. flexor digitorum profundus to first digit
18 Interdigital ligaments

150 Palmar aspect of the manus of the left thoracic limb of a dog. The tendons of the superficial digital flexor muscle have been reflected distally to reveal the tendons of the deep digital flexor muscle. The flexor retinaculum has been removed to show the deep digital flexor tendon running through the carpal canal.

1 Cut edge of the flexor retinaculum
2 Area of carpal canal
3 Tendon of the M. flexor digitorum profundus (cut proximally)
4 Mm. interossei
5 Tendon of M. flexor digitorum superficialis (reflected distally)

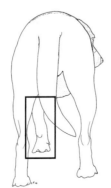

Clinical Note
1 The flexor retinaculum forms the palmar boundary of the carpal canal which in the dog and cat contains the structure **3** but not **5**.

151 Palmar aspect of the manus of the left thoracic limb of a dog. The tendons of the superficial and deep digital flexor muscles have been cut and reflected distally to reveal the vacated carpal canal.

1 Tendon of the M. flexor digitorum superficialis (cut and reflected distally)
2 Tendon of the M. flexor digitorum profundus (cut and reflected distally)
3 Area of carpal canal
4 Palmar carpal fibrocartilage (palmar carpal ligament)
5 Accessory carpal bone
6 Remains of the cut synovial sheath of the tendon of M. flexor digitorum profundus

Clinical Note
4 This plate of fibrocartilage forms the dorsal boundary of the carpal canal.
5 This bone forms the lateral boundary of the carpal canal.

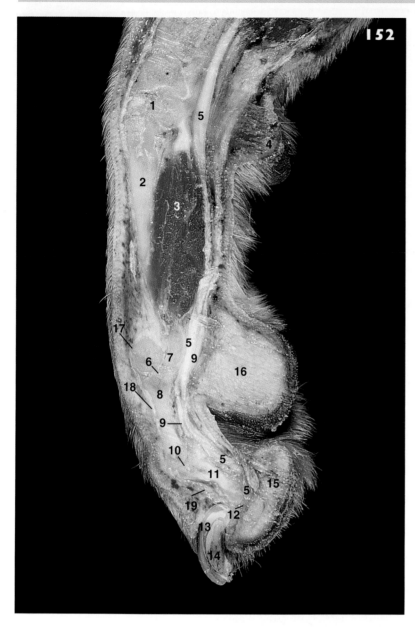

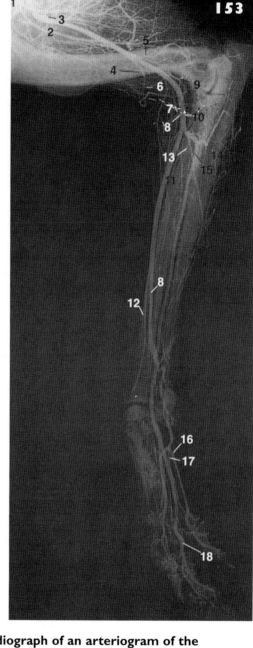

152   Axial section through the carpus and third digit of the manus of a dog.

1 Carpus	10 Proximal interphalangeal joint
2 Third metacarpal bone	11 Middle phalanx
3 M. interosseus	12 Distal interphalangeal joint
4 Carpal pad	13 Claw
5 Tendon of M. flexor digitorum	14 Ungual process of distal phalanx
profundus	15 Digital pad
6 Metacarpophalangeal joint	16 Metacarpal pad
7 Proximal sesamoid	17 Dorsal sesamoid
8 Proximal phalanx	18 Tendon of M. extensor
9 Tendon of M. flexor digitorum	digitorum communis
superficialis	19 Dorsal elastic ligament

153   Mediolateral radiograph of an arteriogram of the thoracic limb of a dog.

1 Axillary artery	10 Common interosseous artery
2 Branchial artery	11 Deep antebrachial artery
3 Deep brachial artery	12 Radial artery
4 Bicipital artery	13 Caudal interosseous artery
5 Colateral ulnar artery	14 Cranial interosseous artery
6 Superficial branchial artery	15 Ulnar artery
7 Transverse cubital artery	16 Palmar common digital arteries
8 Median artery	17 Palmar metacarpal arteries
9 Recurrent ulnar artery	18 Palmar proper digital arteries

Clinical Note

7   This position where the flexor tendons pass over the palmar aspect of the proximal sesamoids is termed the proximal scutum.

9   The lower number **9** is placed where the tendon of the superficial digital flexor forms a tendinous sleeve (manica) to allow the tendon of the deep digital flexor to perforate through it. Immediately distal to the marker the superficial flexor tendon inserts onto the complimentary cartilage of the middle phalanx on the palmar aspect of the proximal interphalangeal joint. This latter cartilaginous structure forms the middle scutum for the flexor tendons.

12   The palmar aspect of the joint is crossed by the tendon of the deep digital flexor and is termed the distal scutum. In the dog a cartilaginous nodule is present in the tendon at this level.

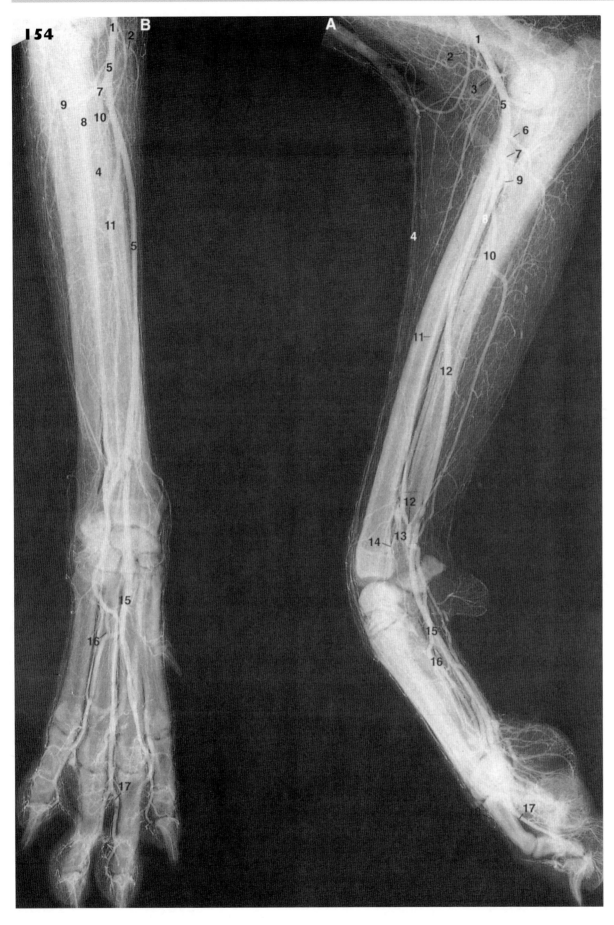

154   Mediolateral (A) and craniocaudal dorsoplantar (B) radiographs of an arteriogram of the thoracic limb of a dog.

1   Brachial artery
2   Superficial brachial artery
3   Transverse cubital artery
4   Cranial superficial antebrachial artery
5   Median artery
6   Recurrent ulnar artery
7   Common interosseous artery
8   Caudal interosseous artery
9   Cranial interosseous artery
10 Ulnar artery
11 Radial artery
12 Anastomosis of the ulnar and caudal interosseous arteries
13 Radial palmar branch
14 Radial dorsal carpal branch
15 Palmar common digital arteries
16 Palmar metacarpal arteries
17 Palmar proper digital arteries
18 Dorsal proper digital arteries

155 Mediolateral radiograph of a venogram of the thoracic limb of a dog.

1 Accessory cephalic vein
2 Cephalic vein
3 Radial vein
4 Interosseous vein
5 Ulnar vein
6 Median vein
7 Median cubital vein
8 Brachial vein
9 Axillobrachial vein
10 Omobrachial vein
11 Axillary vein
12 External jugular vein
13 Internal thoracic vein
14 Precava
15 Cranial vena cava
16 Right side of heart

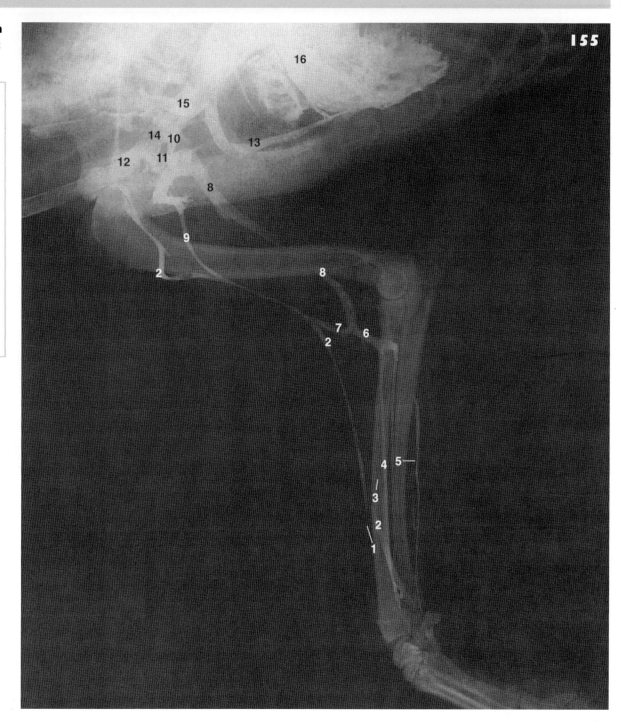

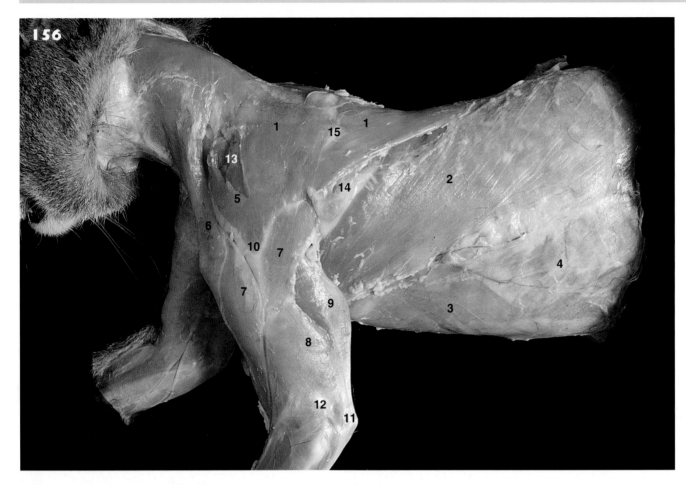

156   A lateral aspect of the shoulder and brachium of the left thoracic limb of a cat.

1	M. trapezius	8	M. triceps brachii (lateral head)
2	M. latissimus dorsi	9	M. triceps brachii (long head)
3	M. pectoralis profundus	10	Acromion
4	M. obliquus externus abdominis	11	Olecranon
5	M. omotransversarius	12	Lateral epicondyle of humerus
6	M. cleidocephalicus, pars cervicalis (M. brachiocephalicus)	13	Superficial cervical lymph nodes
7	M. deltoideus	14	M. serratus ventralis (situated deeply)
		15	Scapula

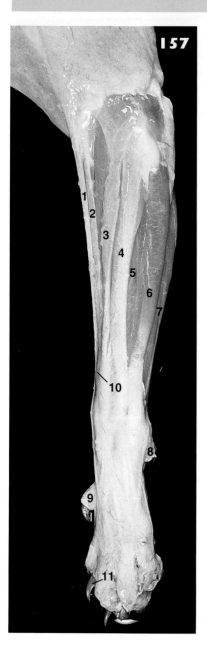

157 Craniolateral aspect of the antebrachium and manus of the left thoracic limb of a cat.

1 Cephalic vein
2 M. brachioradialis
3 M. extensor carpi radialis
4 M. extensor digitorum communis
5 M. extensor digitorum lateralis
6 M. extensor carpi ulnaris (M. ulnaris lateralis)
7 M. flexor carpi ulnaris (ulnar head)
8 Carpal pad
9 First digit (dew claw)
10 M. abductor pollicis longus
11 Claw of third digit

158 Caudomedial aspect of the antebrachium and manus of the left thoracic limb of a cat.

1 Olecranon
2 Medial epicondyle
3 M. flexor carpi ulnaris (ulnar head)
4 M. flexor digitorum superficialis
5 M. flexor digitorum profundus (humeral head)
6 M. flexor carpi radialis
7 M. extensor carpi radialis
8 Cephalic vein
9 Carpal pad
10 First digit (dew claw)
11 Metacarpal pad
12 Digital pad of second digit

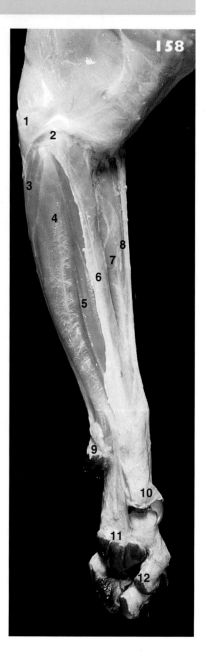

5 THORAX

The osteological features of the thoracic region are revealed using bony specimens and radiographs. With prepared dissections, the musculature is serially displayed from the superficial to the deep layers to reveal the thoracic contents and to demonstrate the topography. The additional technique of B-mode ultrasonography is used to further illustrate cardiac anatomy, and cross-sectional specimens tie together the topographical relationships of the intrathoracic organs.

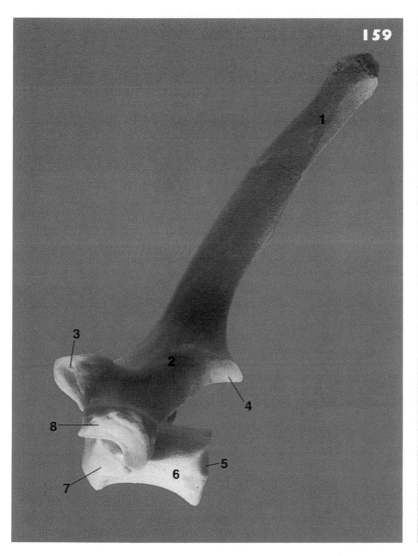

159   Lateral aspect of the first thoracic vertebra of a dog.

1	Spinous process	6	Body
2	Lamina	7	Cranial costal fovea
3	Mamillary process	8	Costal fovea of transverse
4	Caudal articular surface		process
5	Caudal costal fovea		

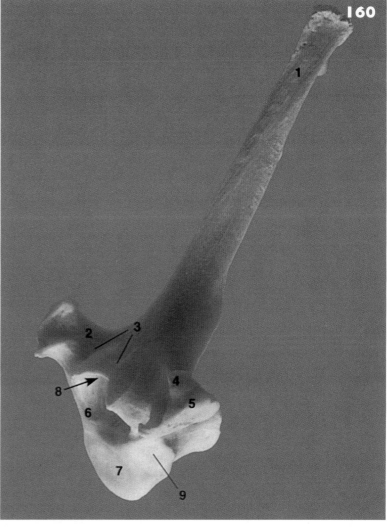

160   Craniolateral aspect of the sixth thoracic vertebra of a dog.

1	Spinous process	6	Pedicle
2	Lamina	7	Body
3	Cranial articular surface	8	Vertebral foramen
4	Transverse process	9	Cranial costal fovea
5	Costal fovea of 4		

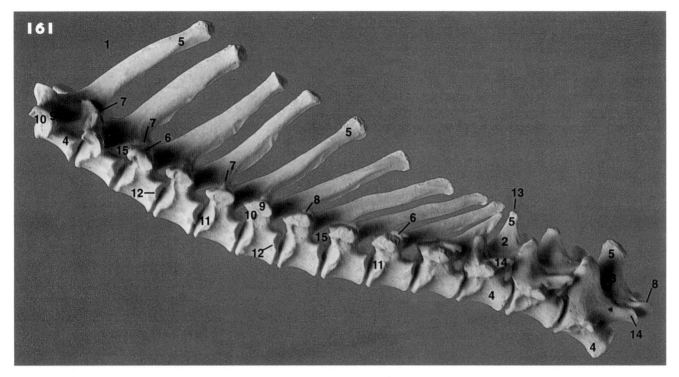

161 Lateral aspect of the articulated thoracic vertebrae of a dog.

1 First ⎫	6 Cranial articular process	11 Cranial costal fovea
2 Eleventh ⎬ thoracic vertebra	7 Mamillary process	12 Caudal costal fovea
3 Thirteenth ⎭	8 Caudal articular process	13 Anticlinal vertebra
4 Body	9 Transverse process	14 Accessory process
5 Spinous process	10 Cranial costal fovea of 9	15 Intervention foramen

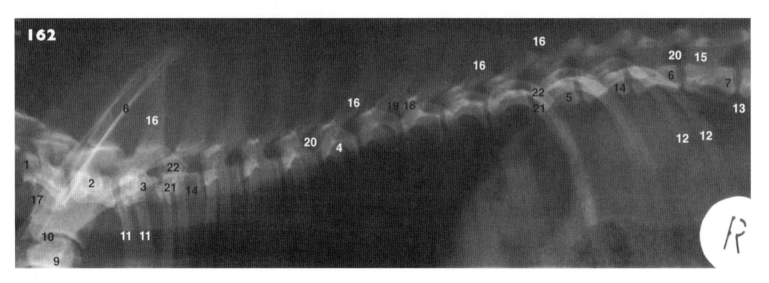

162 Radiograph of the lateral aspect of the thoracic portion of the vertebral column of a dog.

1 Sixth ⎫ cervical vertebra	10 Shoulder joint	17 Transverse process (plate-like
2 Seventh ⎭	11 First ⎫	lamina of sixth cervical
3 First ⎫	12 Twelfth ⎬ rib	vertebra)
4 Sixth ⎪ thoracic	13 Thirteenth (floating) ⎭	18 Cranial articular process
5 Eleventh (anticlinal) ⎬ vertebra	14 Body	19 Caudal articular process
6 Thirteenth ⎭	15 Dorsal and ventral borders of	20 Intervertebral foramina
7 First lumbar vertebra	vertebral foramen (vertebral	21 Head ⎫ of rib
8 Scapula	canal)	22 Tubercle ⎭
9 Humerus	16 Spinous process	

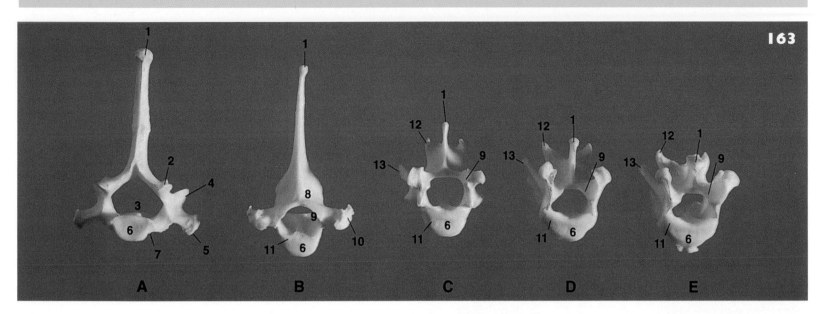

163   Caudal aspect of the first thoracic vertebra (A) and cranial aspect of the sixth (B), eleventh (C), twelfth (D) and thirteenth (E) thoracic vertebrae of a cat.

1 Spinous process	7 Caudal costal fovea
2 Caudal articular surface	8 Lamina
3 Vertebral foramen	9 Cranial articular surface
4 Mamillary process	10 Transverse process
5 Transverse process (with cranial costal fovea)	11 Cranial costal fovea
	12 Caudal articular process
6 Body	13 Accesory process

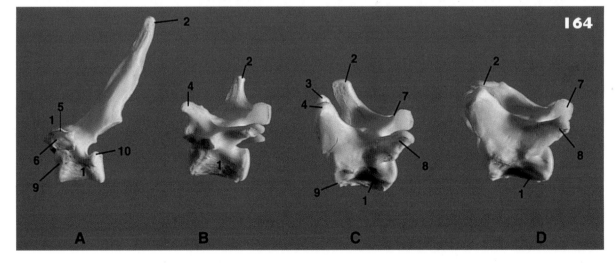

164   Left lateral aspect of the sixth (A), eleventh (anticlinal) (B), twelfth (C) and thirteenth (D) thoracic vertebrae of a cat.

1 Body	6 Costal fovea of 5
2 Spinous process	7 Caudal articular process
3 Cranial articular process	8 Accessory process
4 Mamillary process	9 Cranial costal fovea
5 Transverse process	10 Caudal costal fovea

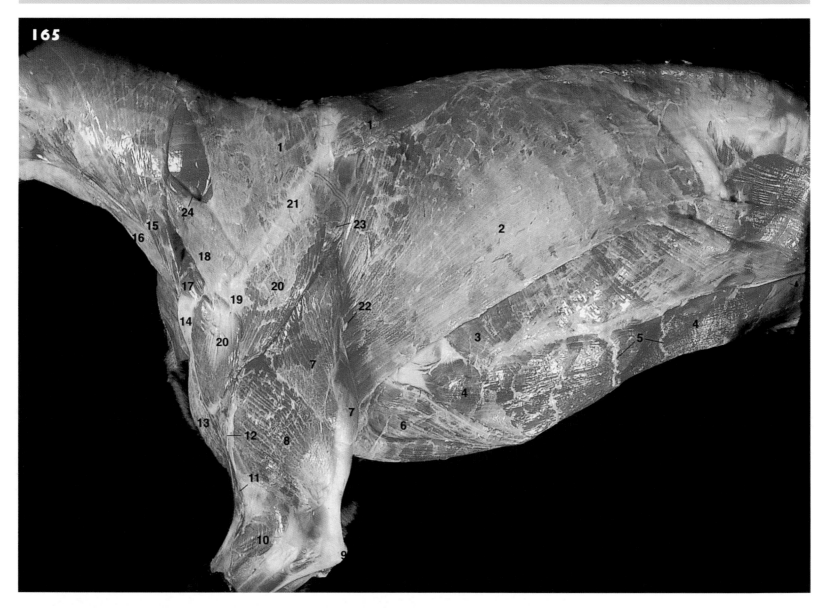

165 Lateral aspect of the superficial muscles of the shoulder and brachium of a dog. The cutaneous trunci and sphincter colli muscles have been removed.

1 M. trapezius	9 Olecranon	17 M. supraspinatus
2 M. latissimus dorsi	10 Extensor group	18 M. omotransversarius
3 M. obliquus externus	11 Cephalic vein	19 Acromion process
abdominis	12 Axillobrachial vein	20 M. deltoideus
4 M. rectus abdominis	13 M. cleidobrachialis	21 Scapular spine
5 Tendinous intersections	14 Greater tubercle of humerus	22 Intercostobrachial nerve
6 M. pectoralis profundus	15 M. cleidocephalicus, pars	(second thoracic nerve)
7 M. triceps brachii (long head)	cervicalis	23 Subscapular artery and vein
8 M. triceps brachii (lateral head)	16 M. sternocephalicus	24 Superficial cervical lymph nodes

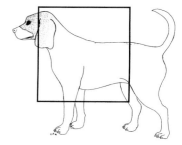

Clinical Note

2 & 3 In a lateral approach to carry out a surgical thoracotomy the M. latissimus dorsi has to be transected across the direction of the muscle fibres. The underlying thoracodorsal nerve may be sectioned by this incision.

9 Note that the olecranon process lies opposite the level of the 5th rib in a standing dog. Thus in order to auscultate or carry out a cardiac ultrasound the limb has to be drawn cranially to examine at the 3rd and 4th intercostal spaces.

24 This lymph node is commonly palpated during routine clinical examination. It is the lymph node directly receiving drainage from the thoracic limb and thus enlargement of this node alone would indicate infection within the ipsilateral thoracic limb.

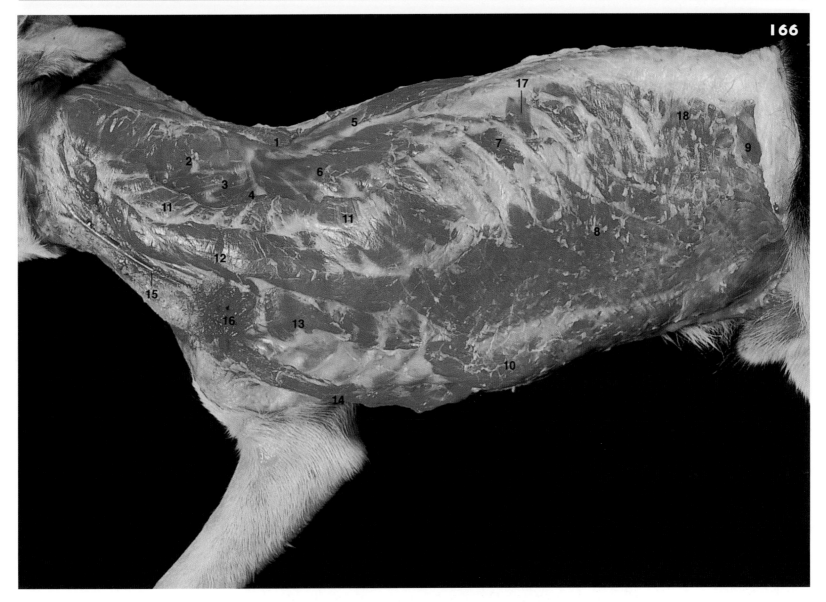

166   Lateral aspect of the muscles of the neck, thorax and abdominal wall of a dog. The left thoracic limb has been moved along with its extrinsic muscles. The axillary vessels and the brachial plexus have been sectioned in the process.

1 M. rhomboideus (cut)	8 M. obliquus externus abdominis, pars costalis	14 Mm. pectorales (cut)
2 M. splenius		15 External jugular vein
3 M. longissimus cervicis	9 M. obliquus externus abdominis, pars lumbalis	16 Axillary vessels (cut)
4 M. longissimus thoracis		17 M. serratus dorsalis caudalis
5 M. spinalis and M. semispinalis thoracis	10 M. rectus abdominis	18 M. obliquus internus abdominis, pars costalis
6 M. serratus dorsalis cranialis	11 M. serratus ventralis (cut)	
7 Mm. intercostales	12 M. scalenus	
	13 M. rectus thoracis	

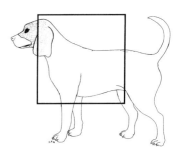

Clinical Note

8 & 11   To achieve entry in to the thorax through an intercostal space during a thoracotomy these muscles have to be parted and held apart with rib retractors. This can be achieved relatively atraumatically by dividing between the pennate attachments to the ribs. Incisions cranial to the 5th intercostal space will necessitate sectioning the M. scalenus (**12**).

167

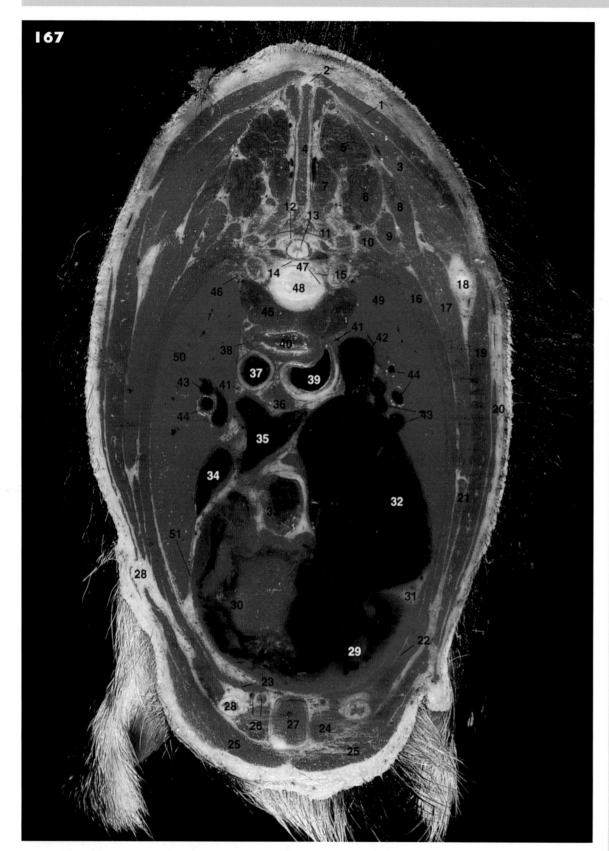

167　Caudal aspect of a transverse section through the trunk of a dog, at the level of the fourth thoracic vertebra.

1	M. trapezius
2	Supraspinous ligament
3	M. rhomboideus
4	Spinous process of fourth thoracic vertebra
5	M. spinalis and M. semispinalis (thoracis and cervicalis)
6	M. longissimus thoracis
7	M. multifidus thoracis
8	M. serratus dorsalis cranialis
9	M. iliocostalis thoracis
10	Mm. rotatores
11	Arch of fourth thoracic vertebra
12	Epidural fat
13	Spinal cord
14	Intercapital ligament
15	Head of rib (caput)
16	Mm. intercostales externi and interni
17	M. serratus ventralis
18	Scapula
19	M. latissimus dorsi
20	M. cutaneus trunci
21	M. scalenus
22	M. rectus abdominis
23	M. transversus thoracis
24	M. intercostalis internus
25	M. pectoralis profundus
26	Internal thoracic artery and vein
27	Sternum
28	Costal cartilage
29	Right ventricle
30	Left ventricle
31	Pericardium overlying coronary vessels in fat of coronary groove
32	Right atrium
33	Left ventricular outflow tract (aortic valve)
34	Left auricle
35	Pulmonary artery (bifurcating)
36	Tracheobronchial lymph node
37	Aorta
38	Thoracic duct
39	Trachea
40	Oesophagus
41	Left and right vagus nerves
42	Right azygos vein
43	Pulmonary veins
44	Bronchi
45	M. longus colli
48	Sympathetic trunk
47	Annulus fibrosus ⎱ of interver-
48	Nucleus pulposus ⎰ tebral disc
49	Cranial lobe of right lung
50	Cranial lobe of left lung
51	Phrenic nerve

Clinical Note
37 & 40　Note that at the level of the base of the heart, the aorta lies to the left of the oesophagus within the mediastinal space. Thus if surgical access to the oesophagus is sought by performing a thoracotomy it is best performed from the right side, to avoid the aorta. In the caudal mediastinal space the oesophagus lies to the left but the aorta is now dorsal and so the surgical approach is performed from the left.

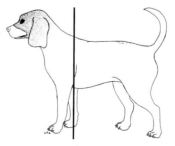

168 Lateral aspect of the left thorax of a dog. The muscles of the thoracic wall and thoracic limb have been resected, along with alternate ribs.

1 M. serratus dorsalis cranialis
2 Brachial plexus
3 Axillary vessels
4 First ⎫
5 Third ⎬ rib
6 Fifth ⎪
7 Thirteenth (floating)) ⎭
8 Pars sternalis ⎫
9 Pars costalis ⎬ of diaphragm
10 Centrum tendineum ⎭
11 Left costodiaphragmatic recess
12 M. obliquus externus abdominis
13 Heart
14 Mediastinal pleura
15 Caudal lobe ⎫ of
16 Caudal part of cranial lobe ⎬ left
17 Cranial part of cranial lobe ⎭ lung
18 Thymus
19 Costochondral joints
20 Costal cartilages
21 Sternum
22 Costal arch

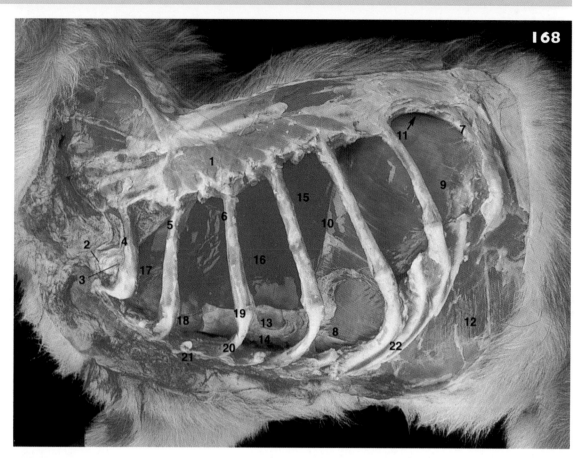

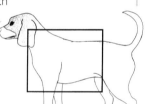

Clinical Note
13 Note that the heart is visible in this position of 3rd, 4th and 5th intercostal space. This aperture in the border of the lung is termed the cardiac notch. It is significant as a window for examination for the purpose of auscultation and echocadiography as there is direct access to the heart without overlying lung field. There is a similar cardiac notch on the right side (see Fig. 169, **15**).

169 Lateral aspect of the opened right thorax of a dog. The right thoracic wall and thoracic limb have been removed, along with alternate ribs.

1 Brachial plexus
2 Intercostal vessels
3 First ⎫
4 Fourth ⎬ rib
5 Eighth ⎪
6 Thirteenth (floating) ⎭
7 Right costodiaphragmatic recess
8 M. obliquus externus abdominis
9 M. obliquus internus abdominis
10 Pars costalis ⎫ of diaphragm
11 Pars sternalis ⎭
12 Caudal lobe ⎫
13 Middle lobe ⎬ of right lung
14 Cranial lobe ⎭
15 Cardiac notch
16 Heart
17 Mediastinal pleura
18 Sternum

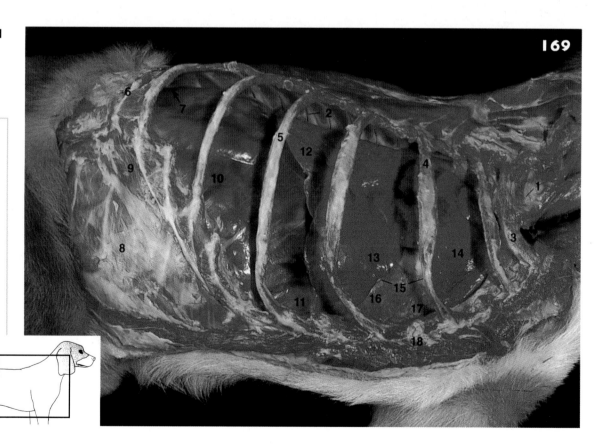

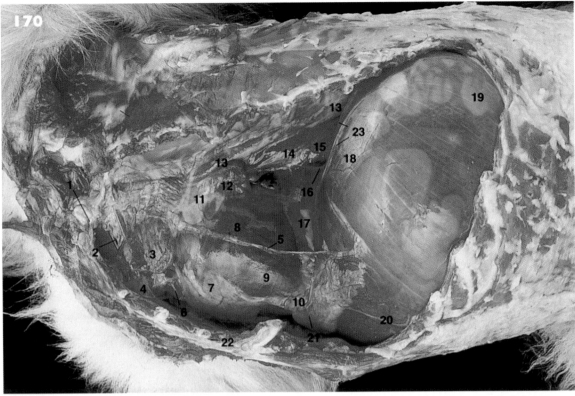

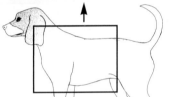

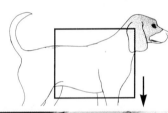

170   Lateral aspect of the opened left thorax of a dog. The left lung has been resected to expose the mediastinum and its contents.

1   Brachial plexus
2   Internal thoracic vein and artery
3   Thymus
4   Mediastinal pleura
5   Phrenic nerve
6   Right auricle
7   Right ventricle
8   Left auricle
9   Left ventricle
10   Apex   } of heart
11   Base
12   Pulmonary (cut) vessels and left bronchus
13   Aorta
14   Oesophagus
15   Dorsal branch   } of vagus
16   Ventral branch   } nerve
17   Accessory lobe of right lung
18   Centrum tendineum
19   Pars costalis   } of diaphragm
20   Pars sternalis
21   Position of sternopericardiac ligament
22   Fifth rib and costal cartilage
23   Hiatus oesophageus

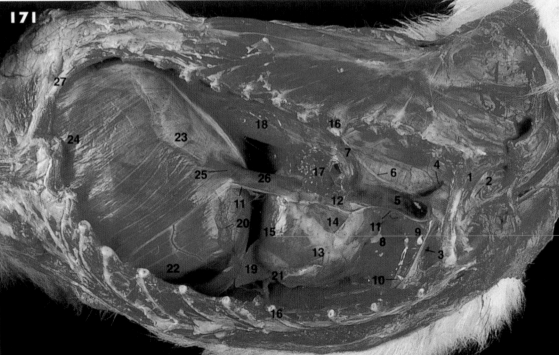

171   Lateral aspect of the opened right thorax of a dog. The right lung has been resected to expose the mediastinum and its contents.

1   First rib
2   Brachial plexus
3   Internal thoracic artery and vein
4   Right costocervical vein
5   Cranial vena cava
6   Vagus nerve (crossing trachea)
7   Right azygos vein
8   Cranial lobe of left lung
9   Thymus
10   Mediastinal pleura
11   Right phrenic nerve
12   Base of heart
13   Right ventricle
14   Right atrium
15   Left ventricle
16   Fifth rib
17   Pulmonary vessels (cut) and bronchus
18   Oesophagus with vagus nerve
19   Left lung
20   Plica venae cavae
21   Apex of heart
22   Pars sternalis   } of diaphragm
23   Centrum tendineum
24   Pars costalis
25   Foramen venae cavae
26   Caudal vena cava
27   Thirteenth (floating) rib

172   Ventral aspect of the opened thorax of a dog. The sternum and costal cartilages have been removed to reveal the thoracic viscera.

1   Larynx with M. cricothyroideus
2   Trachea
3   Thyroid gland
4   M. sternothyroideus
5   M. sternocephalicus
6   Carotid sheath (containing common carotid artery and vagosympathetic trunk)
7   External jugular vein
8   Manubrium sterni
9   Axillary vessels
10 Mediastinal pleura
11 Cranial vena cava
12 Right azygos vein
13 Cranial lobe   ⎫
14 Middle lobe   ⎬ of right lung
15 Caudal lobe   ⎪
16 Accessory lobe   ⎭
17 Cranial part of left lobe ⎫
18 Caudal part of left lobe   ⎬ of left lung
19 Caudal lobe   ⎭
20 Right subclavian artery
21 Left subclavian artery
22 Right atrium
23 Base of heart
24 Right ventricle
25 Pericardium
26 Pulmonary vessels at hilus of lung
27 Caudal vena cava with right phrenic nerve
28 Pars sternalis   ⎫
29 Centrum tendineum   ⎬ of diaphragm
30 Foramen venae cavae
31 Xiphoid process
32 Left ventricle
33 Apex of heart

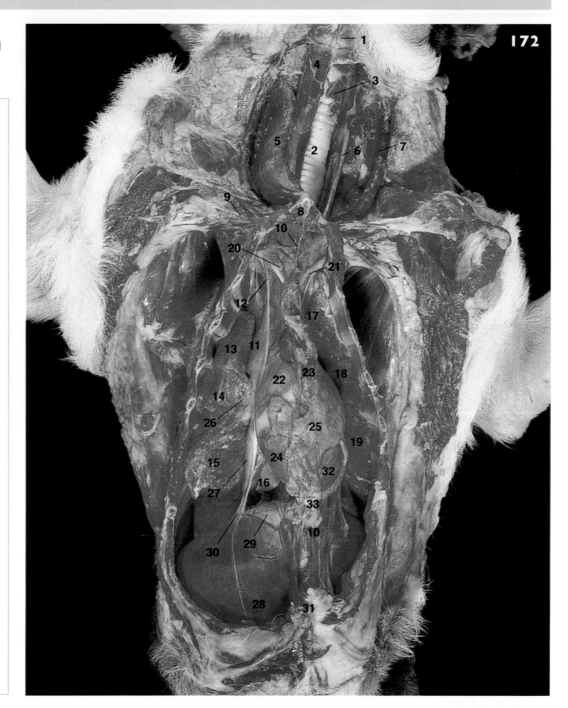

172

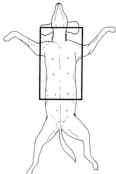

◄— Clinical Note (Fig. 170)
3   The thymus is large in this dog indicating that it is an active organ of an immature animal. As the dog matures the organ declines in activity and thus in size. An older dog would have a small, less obvious organ.
14, 15 & 16   Note the position of the oesophagus as it lies in the caudal mediastinum. This is a common sight for obstruction of the oesophagus by a foreign body and care should be taken when incising the oesophagus to preserve the vagal nerve branches as they lie on the surface of the organ.
23   The hiatus oesophageus is a natural passageway through the diaphragm between the abdominal and thoracic cavities. It is a potential sight for herniation of the diaphragm and may have to be repaired surgically from a left-side thoracotomy incision.

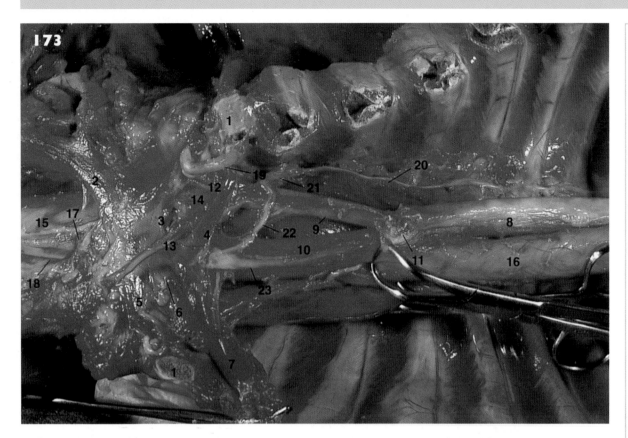

1	First rib
2	Left brachiocephalic vein
3	Left subclavian vein
4	Left costocervical vein
5	Right brachiocephalic vein
6	Internal thoracic vein (cut)
7	Cranial vena cava (cut with artery forceps)
8	Descending aorta
9	Left subclavian artery
10	Brachiocephalic artery
11	Proximal end of aortic arch (cut)
12	Costocervical trunk
13	Internal thoracic artery
14	Continuation of subclavian artery to become axillary artery
15	Cervical oesophagus
16	Thoracic oesophagus
17	Recurrent laryngeal nerve
18	Carotid sheath (containing common carotid artery and vagosympathetic trunk)
19	Vertebral nerve
20	Sympathetic trunk or chain
21	Cervicothoracic ganglion (stellate)
22	Ansa subclavia
23	Left vagus nerve (cut)

173   Exposure of the dorsocranial region of the thorax of a dog. The thoracic viscera have been resected by severing the aortic arch and the venae cavae at the base of the heart.

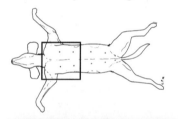

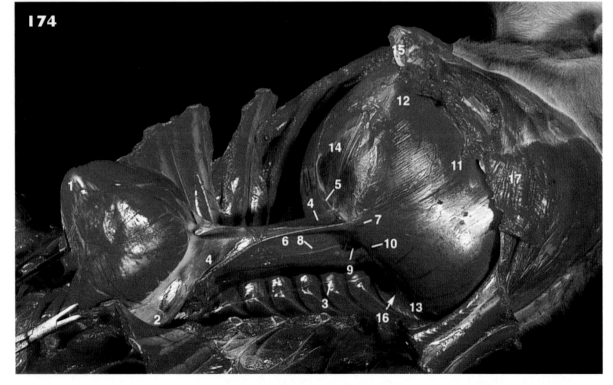

174

1	Apex of heart
2	Cranial vena cava
3	Sympathetic trunk
4	Caudal vena cava
5	Foramen venae cavae
6	Oesophagus
7	Hiatus oesophageus
8	Vagus nerve
9	Aorta
10	Hiatus aorticus
11	Pars costalis
12	Pars sternalis
13	Pars lumbalis } of diaphragm
14	Centrum tendineum
15	Xiphoid process
16	Recessus phrenicolumbalis
17	M. serratus ventralis

174   Cranial aspect of the diaphragm of a dog, viewed from the right. The lungs have been removed and the heart displaced caudally.

175   Paramedian section through the thoracic, abdominal and pelvic cavities of a male dog, showing the topography of the structures of the left side.

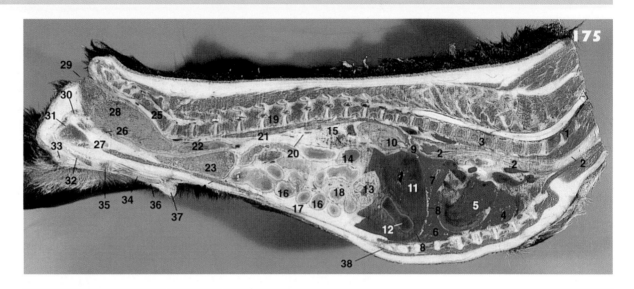

1	Cervical vertebrae	14	Transverse colon	27	Symphysis pelvis
2	Oesophagus	15	Pancreas	28	Rectum
3	Thoracic vertebrae	16	Jejunum	29	Anus
4	Cranial lobe of left lung	17	Greater omentum	30	Root of penis
5	Right ventricle	18	Great mesentery	31	Corpus cavernosum penis
6	Accessory lobe of right lung	19	Lumbar vertebrae	32	Body of penis
7	Caudal lobe of left lung	20	Aorta	33	Testis
8	Diaphragm	21	M. psoas major	34	Glans penis
9	Hiatus oesophageus	22	Descending colon	35	Bulbus glandis
10	Cardiac region of stomach	23	Urinary bladder	36	Pars longa glandis
11	Liver	24	M. rectus abdominis	37	Prepuce
12	Gall bladder	25	Sacrum	38	Xiphoid process of sternum
13	Pyloric region of stomach	26	Prostate		

176   Paramedian section through the thoracic, abdominal and pelvic cavities of a male dog, showing the topography of the structures of the right side.

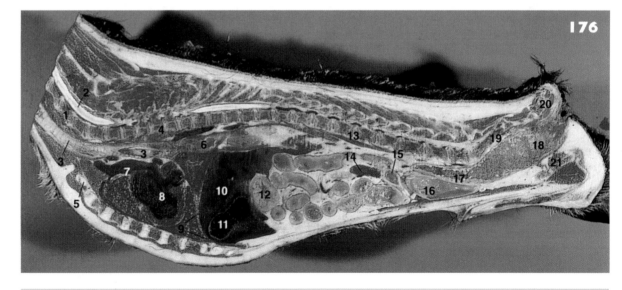

1	Cervical vertebrae	8	Right ventricle	15	Transverse duodenum
2	Spinal cord	9	Diaphragm	16	Urinary bladder
3	Trachea	10	Liver	17	Descending colon
4	Thoracic vertebrae	11	Gall bladder	18	Rectum
5	Manubrium sterni	12	Stomach	19	Sacrum
6	Oeosphagus	13	Lumbar vertebrae	20	Caudal vertebrae
7	Cranial vena cava	14	Mesenteric lymph node	21	Symphysis of pubis

177

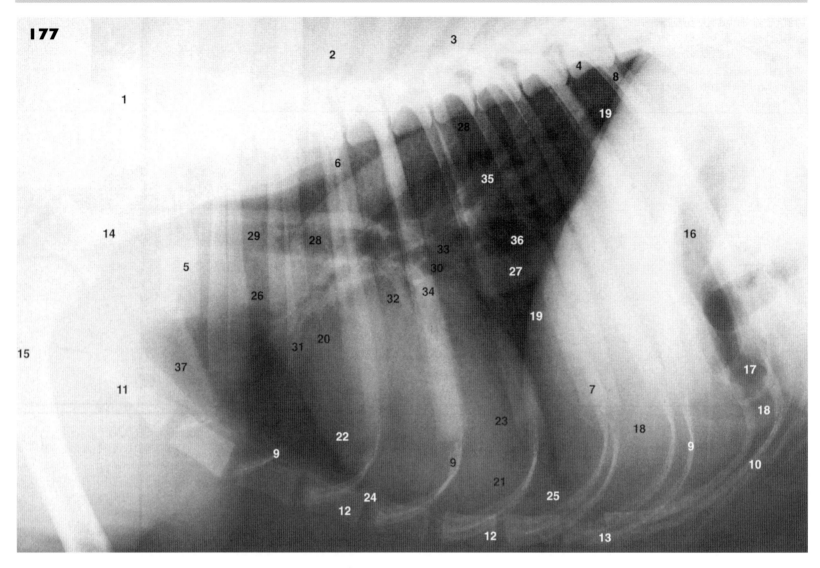

177   Radiograph of the thoracic region of a dog in lateral recumbency.

1	First	} thoracic	14	Scapula
2	Fourth		15	Humerus
3	Seventh	vertebra	16	Stomach
4	Tenth	}	17	Small Intestine
5	First	}	18	Liver
6	Fourth	} rib	19	Diaphragm
7	Seventh		20	Base
8	Tenth	}	21	Apex
9	Costal cartilage		22	Right side
10	Costal arch		23	Left side
11	Manubrium sterni		24	Pericardium
12	Sternebrae		25	Sternopericardiac ligament
13	Xiphoid process		26	Cranial vena cava

27 Caudal vena cava
28 Aorta
29 Trachea
30 Tracheal bifurcation
31 Bronchus to cranial } lobe of
32 Bronchus to middle } lung
33 Bronchus to caudal }
34 Bronchus to accessory lobe of right lung
35 Dorsal bronchi
36 Ventral bronchi
37 Pleural cupula

20 Base
21 Apex } of heart
22 Right side
23 Left side

178   Ventrodorsal radiograph of the thoracic region of a dog.

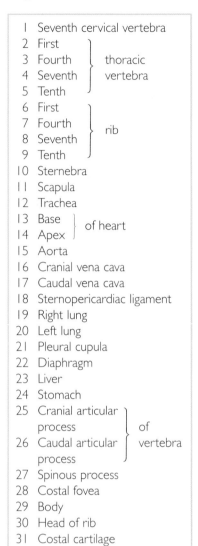

1   Seventh cervical vertebra
2   First   ⎫
3   Fourth ⎬ thoracic
4   Seventh ⎭ vertebra
5   Tenth
6   First   ⎫
7   Fourth ⎬ rib
8   Seventh ⎭
9   Tenth
10 Sternebra
11 Scapula
12 Trachea
13 Base ⎫ of heart
14 Apex ⎭
15 Aorta
16 Cranial vena cava
17 Caudal vena cava
18 Sternopericardiac ligament
19 Right lung
20 Left lung
21 Pleural cupula
22 Diaphragm
23 Liver
24 Stomach
25 Cranial articular ⎫
    process   ⎬ of
26 Caudal articular ⎭ vertebra
    process
27 Spinous process
28 Costal fovea
29 Body
30 Head of rib
31 Costal cartilage

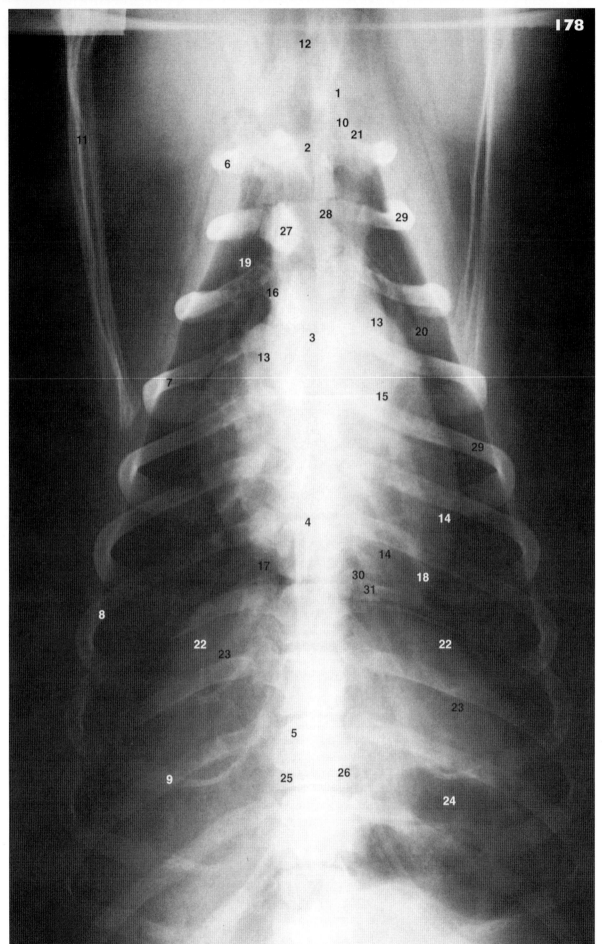

178

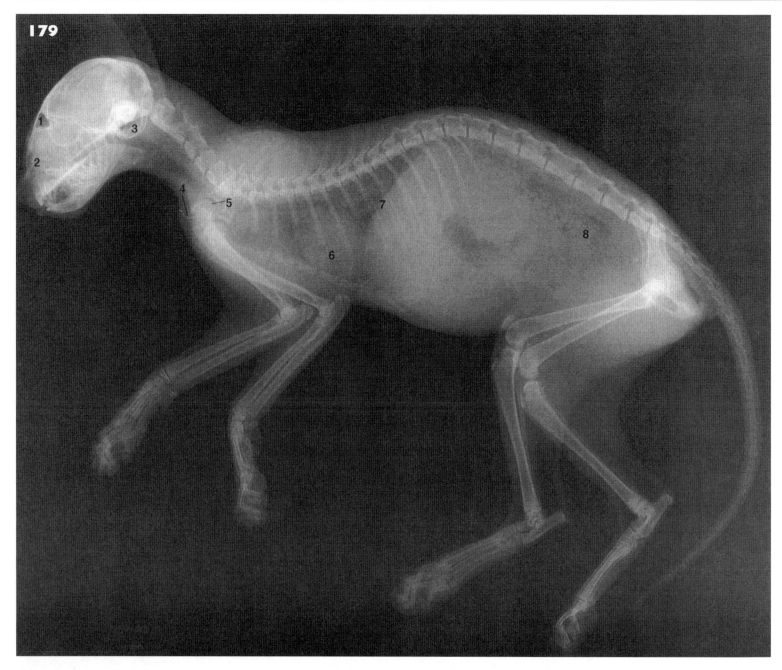

179   Lateral radiograph of a kitten, showing the skeletal elements and centres of ossification.

1 Frontal sinus
2 Maxilla
3 Tympanic bulla
4 Clavicle
5 Suprahamate process on acromion of scapula
6 Heart
7 Diaphragm
8 Descending colon

Clinical Note
4 & 5   The clavicle and the suprahamate process are not found in the dog.
Note the foreshortened facial region of the skull

180 **Dorsoventral radiograph of the head, neck and thorax of a cat.**

1	Canine teeth	11	Suprahamate process
2	Maxilla	12	Clavicle
3	Zygomatic arch	13	Humerus
4	Mandible	14	Olecranon of ulna
5	Tympanic bulla	15	Radius
6	First cervical vertebra (atlas)	16	Apex } of heart
7	Second cervical vertebra (axis)	17	Base }
8	Manubrium sterni	18	Diaphragm
9	First rib	19	First lumbar vertebra
10	Scapula	20	Left } renal outline
		21	Right }

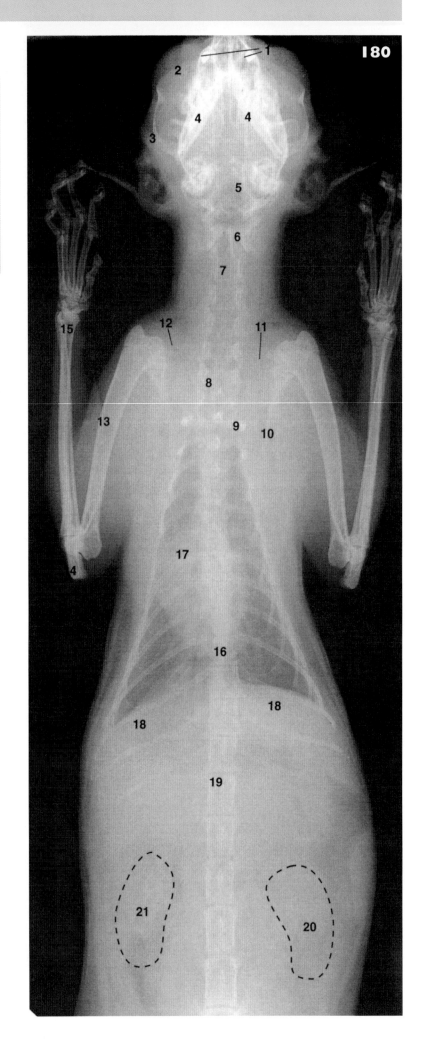

181

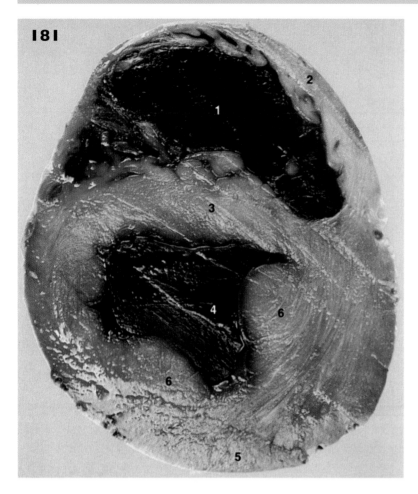

181 Cross section through the ventricles of a dog heart.

1 Lumen } of right ventricle
2 Free wall
3 Interventricular septum
4 Lumen } of left ventrical
5 Free wall
6 Papillary muscles

Clinical Note
This section through the ventricles gives an anatomical plane similar to that in a short-axis ultrasound scan. It is the preferred position for measuring ventricular dimensions with M-mode ultrasonography.

182

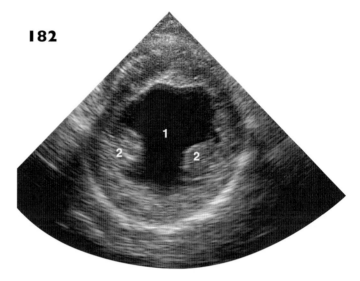

182 Ultrasound scan of a short-axis cross section through the left ventricle of the heart of a dog. The papillary muscles are seen at the periphery of the ventricle.

1 Left ventricle   2 Papillary muscles

183

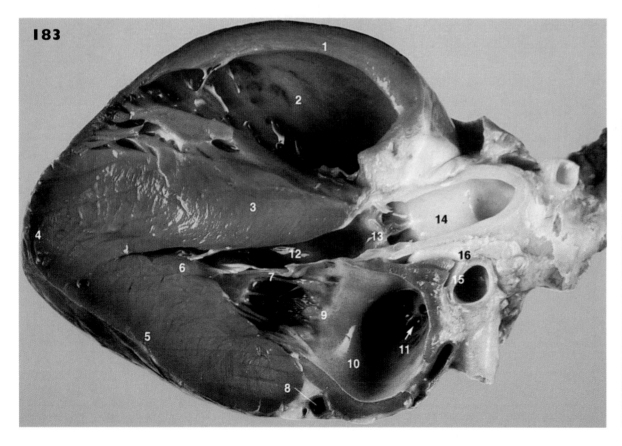

183 Longitudinal section of the heart of a dog, showing the intracardiac structures seen on long-axis ultrasound scans.

1 Free wall } of right
2 Lumen   } ventricle
3 Interventricular septum
4 Apex of heart
5 Free wall of left ventricle
6 Papillary muscle
7 Chordae tendineae
8 Coronary vessels
9 Mitral (left atrioventricular) valve
10 Left atrium
11 Left auricle
12 Outflow tract of left ventricle
13 Aortic valve
14 Aorta
15 Pulmonary artery
16 Base of heart

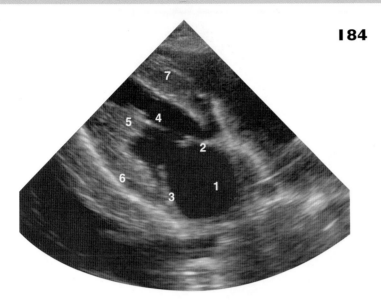

184

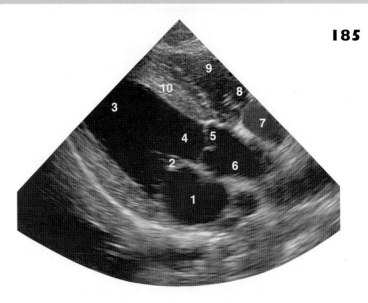

185

184   Ultrasound scan of the left ventricle of the heart of a dog, taken from the left thoracic wall. The plane of the scan is in the long axis.

1	Left atrium	4	Chordae tendineae
2	Septal cusp	5	Papillary muscle in left ventricle
3	Parietal (free wall) cusp	6	Free wall of left ventricle
	} of mitral (left atrioventricular) valve	7	Interventricular septum

185   Ultrasound scan of the heart of a dog, taken from the right side of the thorax. The two atrioventricular valves and the aortic valve are displayed. The plane of the scan is in the long axis.

1	Left atrium	6	Aorta
2	Mitral (left atrioventricular) valve	7	Right atrium
3	Left ventricle	8	Tricuspid (right atrioventricular) valve
4	Outflow tract of 3	9	Right ventricle
5	Aortic valve	10	Interventricular septum

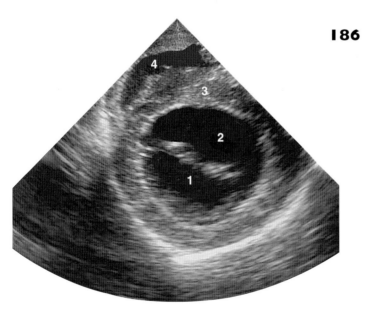

186

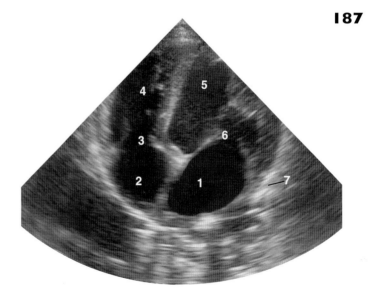

187

186   Right parasternal short-axis (fish mouth) view at level of mitral valve.

1	Parietal (free wall) cusp	3	Interventricular septum
2	Septal cusp	4	Right ventricle
	} of mitral (left) atrioventricular valve		

187   Suprasternal four-chamber view of heart

1	Left atrium	4	Right ventricle
2	Right atrium	5	Left ventricle
3	Tricuspid (left atrioventricular) valve	6	Mitral (left atrioventricular) valve
		7	Pericardium

188

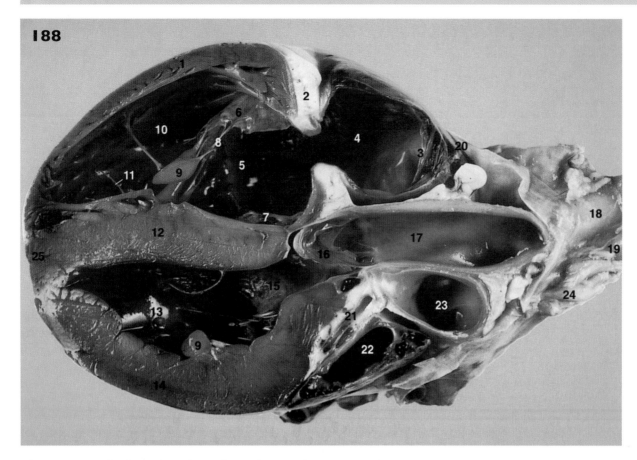

188   Longitudinal section through the heart of a dog, showing the right side and the outflow tract of the left ventricle.

1	Free wall of right ventricle	13	Lumen	} of left ventricle
2	Coronary groove	14	Free wall	
3	Right auricle	15	Outflow tract	
4	Right atrium	16	Aortic valve	
5	Tricuspid (right atrioventricular) valve	17	Aorta	
6	Parietal (free wall) cusp	18	Brachiocephalic trunk	
7	Septal cusp	19	Left subclavian artery	
8	Chordae tendineae	20	Pericardium (cut)	
9	Papillary muscle	21	Coronary vessels	
10	Lumen of right ventricle	22	Left auricle	
11	Trabecula septormarginalis	23	Pulmonary trunk	
12	Interventricular septum	24	Base	} of heart
		25	Apex	

189   Dorsal aspect of the base of the heart of a dog, sectioned to reveal the valvular structures. The atria and auricles have been exposed, and the venae cavae and pulmonary veins removed. Cranial (Cr) and caudal (Ca) orientation are indicated.

1   Right auricle
2   Mm. pectinati
3   Right atrium
4   Tricuspid (right atrioventricular) valve
5   Coronary groove
6   Opening of coronary sinus
7   Fossa ovalis
8   Intervenous tubercle
9   Left atrium
10 Left auricle
11 Mitral (left atrioventricular) valve
12 Right semilunar valvula ⎫
13 Left semilunar valvula ⎬ of aortic valve
14 Dorsal semilunar valvula ⎭
15 Opening for right coronary artery from right sinus of aorta
16 Aorta
17 Pulmonary trunk
18 Conus arteriosus
19 Wall of right ventricle

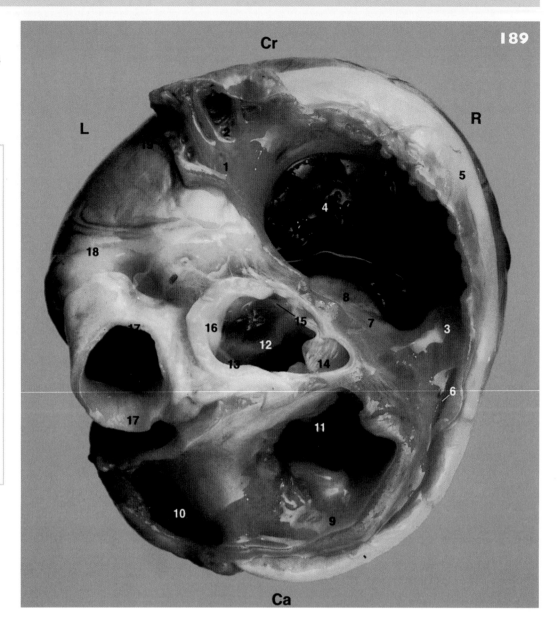

190   Ultrasound scan of the right side of the heart of a dog, taken at the left thoracic wall. The apex of the heart is at the top of the scan.

1   Aortic valve
2   Left atrium
3   Right atrium
4   Tricuspid (right atrioventricular) valve
5   Right ventricle

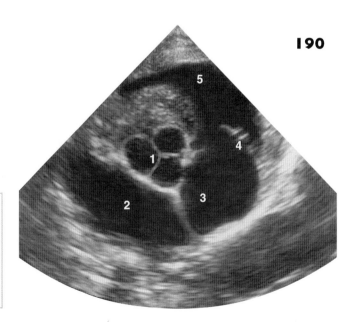

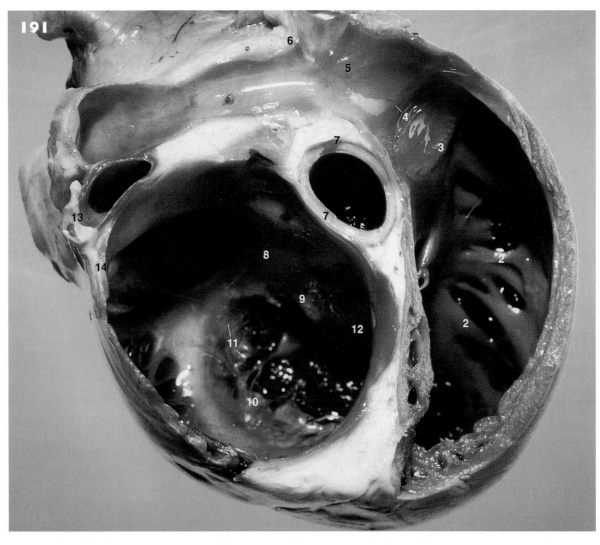

Clinical Note
4 & 5 Note that the pulmonary trunk curls around the aorta so that the two structures are at right angle to each other. This is the scanning field used to interrogate the pulmonary valve in echocardiography. If the aorta is imaged in short axis (cross section) then the pulmonary valve will appear in long axis (longitudinally).

191   Oblique cross section through the heart of a dog, made at the level of the pulmonary valve to show the relationship with the aorta.

1 Free wall of right ventricle	6 Bifurcation of 5	10 Parietal (free wall) cusp
2 Trabeculae carneae	7 Aorta	11 Chordae tendineae
3 Outflow tract of right ventricle	8 Right atrium	12 Right ventricle
4 Pulmonary valve	9 Tricuspid (right atrioventricular)	13 Pulmonary vein
5 Pulmonary artery	valve	14 Right auricle

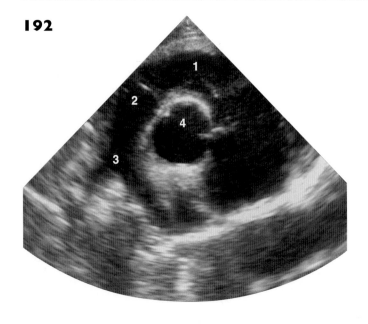

192   Ultrasound scan of the pulmonary valve of the heart of a dog, taken from the left thoracic wall. The pulmonary trunk can be seen curling around the aorta.

1 Outflow tract of right ventricle	3 Pulmonary artery
2 Pulmonary valve	4 Aortic valve

6 ABDOMEN AND PELVIC REGION

The bony framework of the abdominal and pelvic regions is first demonstrated before the layers of soft tissue structures have been exposed. The internal viscera of these regions are then comprehensively displayed using dissected and cross-sectional specimens, radiography and B-mode ultrasonography. Variations between the male and female organs including the external genitalia, are exhibited. Particular attention is paid to the topographical features of the abdomen and the pelvic cavities.

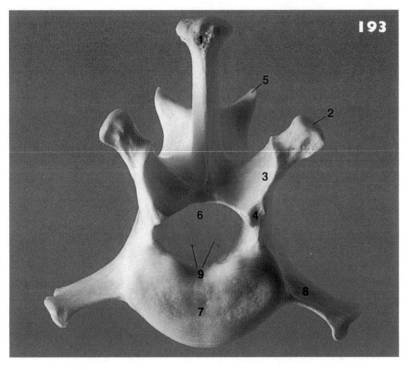

193   Cranial aspect of the first lumbar vertebra of a dog.

1	Spinous process	6	Vertebral foramen
2	Mamillary process	7	Body
3	Cranial articular surface	8	Transverse process
4	Cranial articular process	9	Dorsal foramina
5	Caudal articular process		

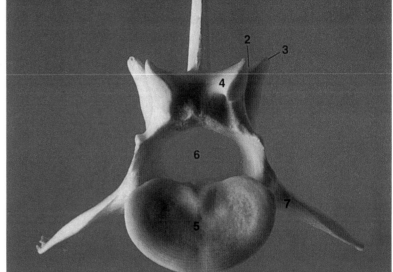

194   Caudal aspect of the fifth lumbar vertebra of a dog.

1	Spinous process	5	Body
2	Cranial articular process	6	Vertebral foramen
3	Mamillary process	7	Transverse process
4	Caudal articular process		

195   Lateral aspect of the sacrum of a dog.

1	Median sacral crest	5	Caudal articular process
2	Intermediate sacral crest	6	Body
3	Wing	7	Transverse process
4	Auricular surface		

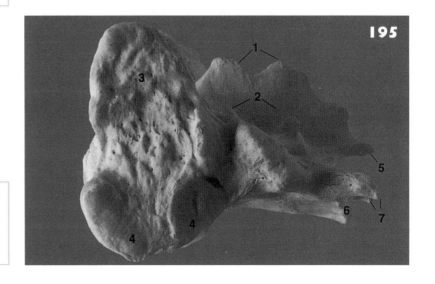

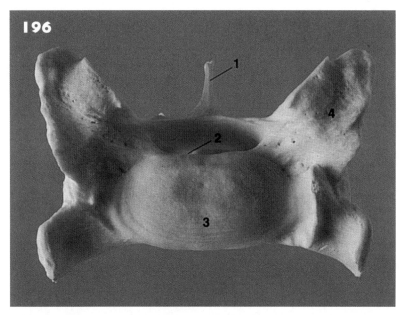

196   Cranial aspect of the sacrum of a dog.

1 Spinous process of median sacral crest	3 Base
2 Sacral canal	4 Wing

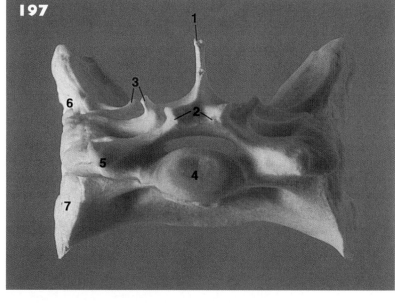

197   Caudal aspect of the sacrum of a dog.

1 Spinous process of median sacral crest	4 Body
2 Caudal articular process	5 Lateral sacral crest
3 Intermediate sacral crest	6 Wing
	7 Auricular surface

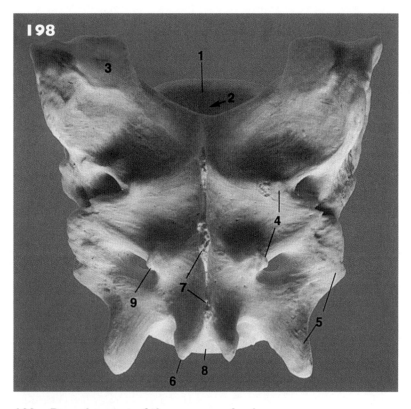

198   Dorsal aspect of the sacrum of a dog.

1 Base	6 Caudal articular process
2 Sacral canal	7 Median sacral crest
3 Cranial articular surface	8 Apex
4 Intermediate sacral crest	9 Dorsal sacral foramina
5 Lateral sacral crest	

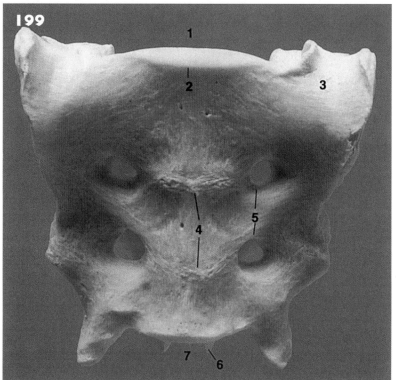

199   Ventral aspect of the sacrum of a dog.

1 Base	5 Pelvic sacral foramina
2 Promontory	6 Caudal articular process
3 Wing	7 Apex
4 Transverse lines	

200 **Dorsal aspect of the fifth caudal vertebra (A), ventral aspect of the fourth (B) and sixth (C) caudal vertebra, and dorsal aspect of the fourteenth caudal vertebra (D) of a dog.**

1　Cranial articular process
2　Mamillary process
3　Neural arch
4　Caudal articular process
5　Transverse process
6　Haemal arch
7　Body
8　Cranial transverse process

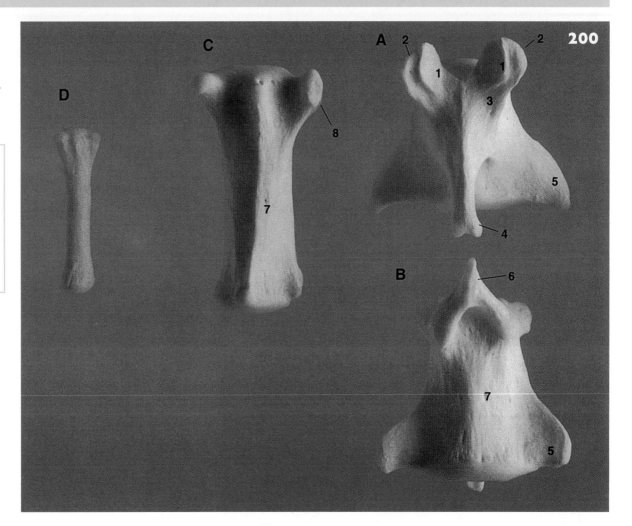

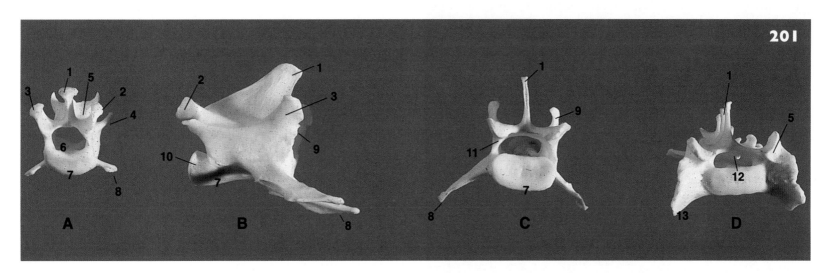

201 **Cranial aspect of the first lumbar vertebra (A), lateral (right side) aspect of the fifth lumbar vertebra (B), caudal aspect of the seventh lumbar vertebra (C), and cranial aspect of the sacrum of a cat.**

1　Spinous process	6　Vertebral foramen	11　Caudal articular surface
2　Caudal articular process	7　Body	12　Sacral canal
3　Mamillary process	8　Transverse process	13　Sacral wing
4　Accessory process	9　Cranial articular process	
5　Cranial articular surface	10　Caudal vertebral notch	

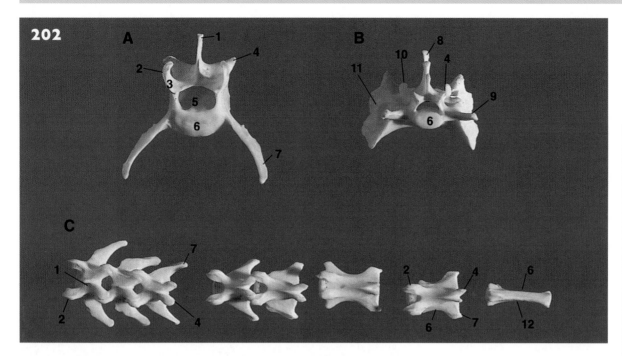

202   Cranial aspect of the seventh lumbar vertebra (A), caudal aspect of the sacrum (B), and dorsal aspect of the first, second, and third caudal vertebrae (C) of a cat.

1	Spinous process
2	Cranial articular process
3	Cranial articular surface
4	Caudal articular process
5	Vertebral foramen
6	Body
7	Transverse process
8	Spinous processes (median sacral crest)
9	Lateral crest
10	Intermediate sacral crest
11	Wing
12	Distal segment of caudal vertebra (dorsal)

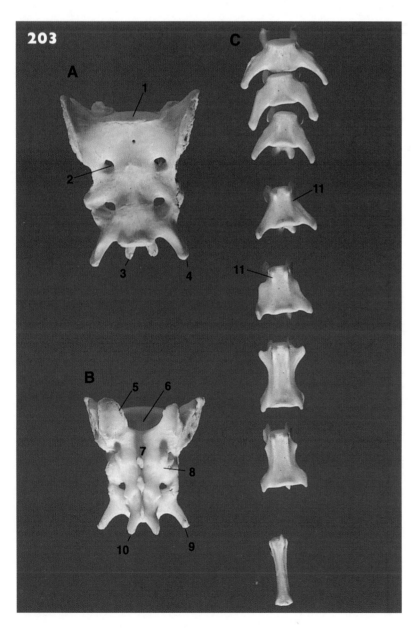

203   Ventral (A) and dorsal aspect (B) of the sacrum, and ventral aspect (C) of several caudal vertebrae of a cat.

1	Promontory	6	Sacral canal
2	Pelvic sacral foramina	7	Median sacral crest
3	Caudal articular surface	8	Intermediate sacral crest
4	Transverse process of lateral sacral crest	9	Lateral sacral crest
5	Cranial articular surface	10	Caudal articular process
		11	Haemal process

204 Lateral aspect of the articulated lumbar vertebrae of a dog.

1	First lumbar vertebra
2	Seventh lumbar vertebra
3	Body
4	Spinous process
5	Cranial articular process
6	Mamillary process
7	Caudal articular process
8	Transverse process
9	Accessory process
10	Intervertebral foramen

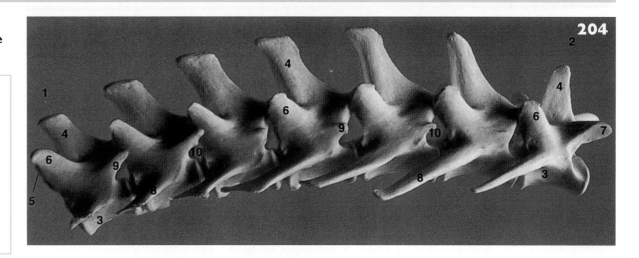

205 Dorsal aspect of the articulated lumbar vertebrae of a dog.

1	First lumbar vertebra
2	Seventh lumbar vertebra
3	Spinous process
4	Cranial articular process
5	Mamillary process
6	Caudal articular process
7	Transverse process
8	Accessory process

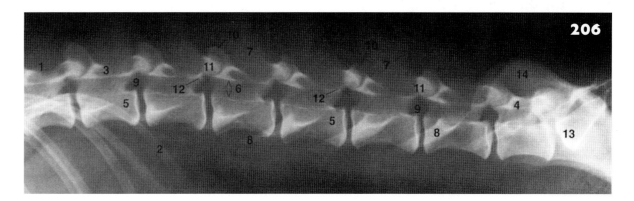

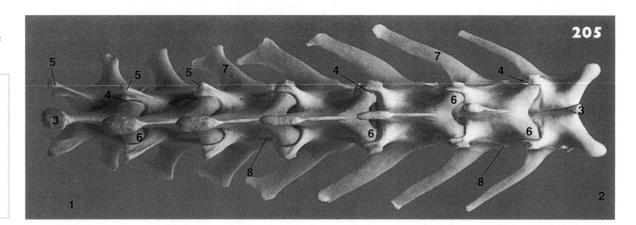

206 Radiograph of the lateral aspect of the lumbar region of the vertebral column of a dog.

1	Thirteenth thoracic vertebra	8	Transverse process of lumbar vertebra
2	Thirteenth (floating) rib		
3	First ⎫ lumbar vertebra	9	Intervertebral foramina
4	Seventh ⎭	10	Cranial articular process
5	Body of vertebra	11	Caudal articular process
6	Dorsal and ventral borders of vertebral foramen (vertebral canal)	12	Accessory process
		13	Body of sacrum
		14	Wing of ilium
7	Spinous process		

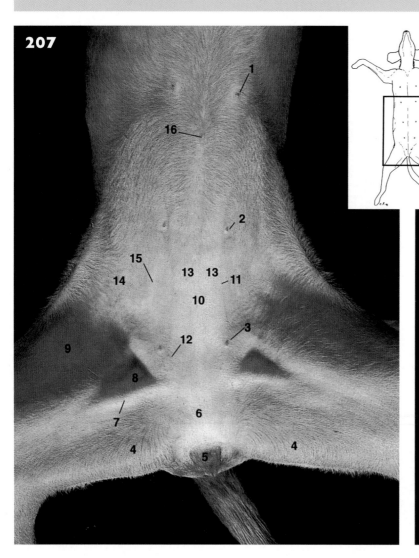

207   Ventral aspect of the intact abdominal wall and inguinal region of a nulliparous bitch.

1	Teat of cranial abdominal	}	
2	Teat of caudal abdominal	} mammary gland	
3	Teat of inguinal abdominal	}	
4	M. gracilis		
5	Vulva		
6	Symphysis pelvis		
7	M. pectineus		
8	Femoral triangle		
9	M. sartorius		
10	Median raphe over linea alba		
11	Caudal superficial epigastric artery and vein		
12	Level of superficial ring of inguinal canal		
13	M. rectus abdominis		
14	M. obliquus externus abdominis and M. obliquus internus abdominis		
15	Lateral border of sheath of M. rectus abdominis		
16	Umbilical scar		

208   Ventral aspect of the intact thoracic, abdominal and inguinal regions of a pregnant bitch.

1	Cranial thoracic	}	
2	Caudal thoracic	}	
3	Cranial abdominal	} mammary gland	
4	Caudal abdominal	}	
5	Inguinal	}	
6	Level of xiphoid process of sternum		
7	Umbilical scar		
8	Teat with orifices		
9	Median raphe overlying linea alba		
10	Vulva		

Clinical Note

1–3 & 1–5   It is of importance to know the direction of flow of the lymphatic drainage from the mammary glands when examining these glands for spread of infection or tumour formation. The cranial and caudal abdominal glands drain to the sternal or axillary lymphocentres. The caudal abdominal and inguinal glands drain to the inguinal lymphocentres, therefore drainage from the cranial abdominal gland may travel both cranially and caudally.

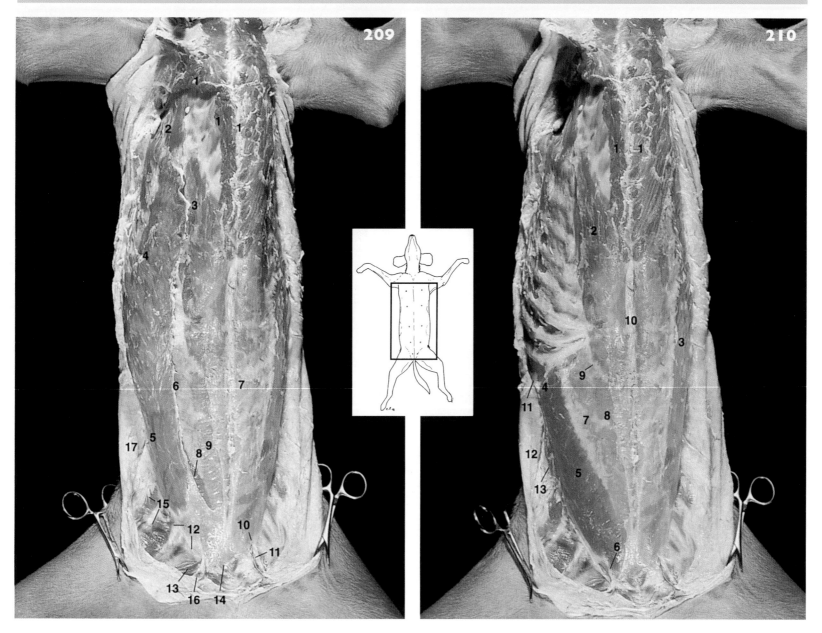

209 Ventral aspect of the thoracic and abdominal regions of a dog. The skin has been removed and the deep pectoral muscle reflected to reveal the muscles of the abdominal wall.

1	M. pectoralis profundus
2	M. scalenus
3	M. rectus abdominis
4	Pars costalis ⎫ of M. obliquus
5	Pars lumbalis ⎬ externus
6	Aponeurosis ⎭ abdominis
	(cut edge)
7	Sheath of M. rectus abdominis
8	M. obliquus internus abdominis
9	Contribution of 6 running in superficial sheath of M. rectus abdominis
10	External inguinal ring
11	Vaginal process with external pudendal vessels
12	Femoral triangle
13	M. pectineus
14	Prepubic tendon
15	M. sartorius
16	Superficial inguinal lymph node
17	Reflected skin

210 Ventral aspect of the thoracic and abdominal regions of a dog. The deep pectoral and external oblique abdominal muscles have been removed on the right side to reveal the internal oblique abdominal muscles.

1	M. pectoralis profundus
2	M. rectus abdominis
3	M. obliquus externus abdominis
4	Pars costalis ⎫ of M.
5	Pars abdominis ⎬ obliquus
6	Pars inguinalis ⎪ internus
	(from inguinal ⎪ abdominis
	ligament) ⎭
7	M. transversus abdominis seen through aponeurosis of M. obliquus internus abdominis
8	Aponeurosis of M. obliquus internus abdominis in superficial sheath of M. rectus abdominis
9	Aponeurosis of M. obliquus internus abdominis running deep to M. rectus abdominis
10	Linea alba
11	Thirteenth (floating) rib
12	Reflected skin
13	M. obliquus externus abdominis (cut edge)

Clinical Note

10 To gain surgical access to the abdominal cavity, incisions are made precisely in the midline ventrally, through the linea alba. Using the linea alba as a portal for entry minimises haemorrhage and provides a sound tissue base for insertion of sutures.

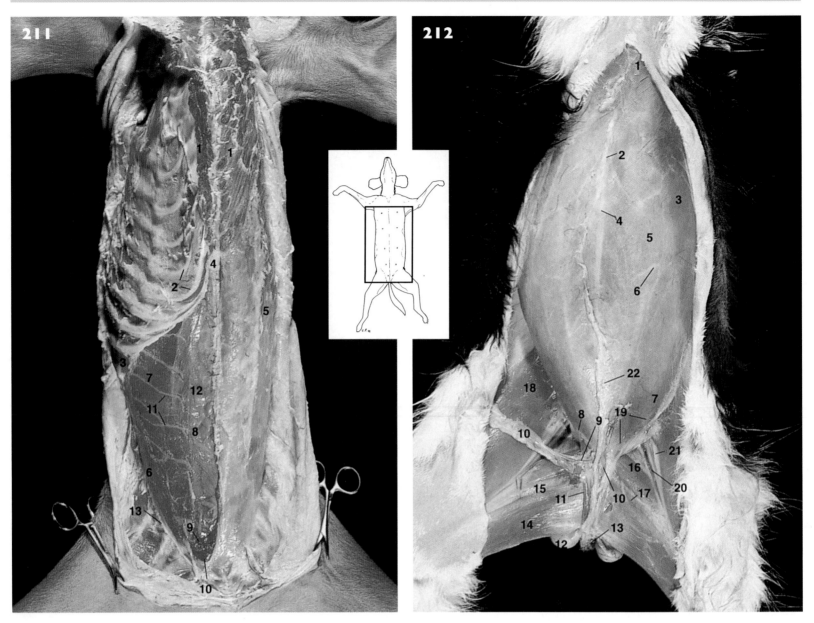

211   Ventral aspect of the thoracic and abdominal regions of a dog. The deep pectoral, external and internal oblique abdominal, and rectus muscles have been removed on the right side to reveal the deeper layers.

1 M. pectoralis profundus	10 M. rectus abdominis (cut
2 Costal cartilages	edge)
3 Thirteenth rib (floating)	11 Medial branches of ventral
4 Xiphoid process of sternum	divisions of thoracic and
5 M. obliquus externus abdominis	lumbar nerves
6 Pars lumbalis ⎫	12 Abdominal viscera seen
7 Pars costalis ⎪	through aponeurosis of 6 and
8 Aponeurosis ⎬ of M.	7, fascia transversalis and
lying deep to ⎪ transversus	parietal peritoneum
10 (resected) ⎪ abdominis	13 M. obliquus internus
9 Aponeurosis lying ⎭	abdominis (cut edge)
superficial to 10	

212   Ventral aspect of the superficial abdominal muscles of a male cat.

1 M. pectoralis profundus	10 Chain of superficial inguinal
2 Linea alba	lymph nodes
3 M. obliquus externus	11 Spermatic cord
abdominis	12 Testis
4 Umbilical scar	13 Prepuce
5 Superficial sheath ⎫ of M.	14 M. gracilis
6 Tendinous ⎬ rectus	15 M. adductor
inscriptions ⎭ abdominis	16 M. pectineus
7 M. obliquus internus abdominis	17 Branch of obturator nerve
seen through aponeurotic	18 M. sartorius
sheet of M. obliquus externus	19 Femoral triangle
abdominus	20 Femoral artery and vein
8 External inguinal ring	21 Saphenous nerve (branch of
9 External pudendal artery and	femoral nerve)
vein	22 Subcutaneous fat

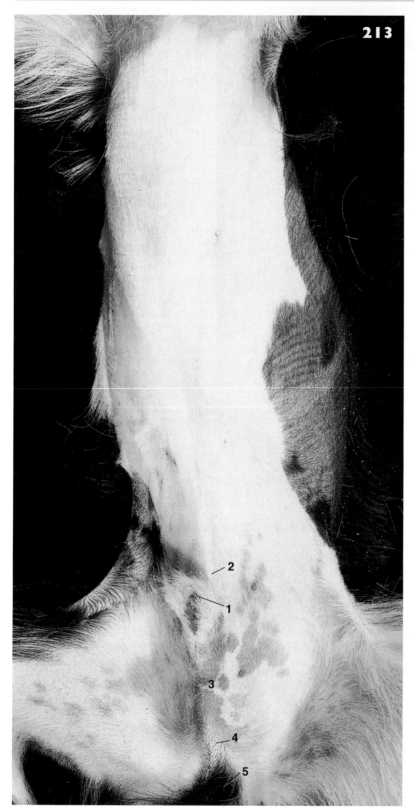

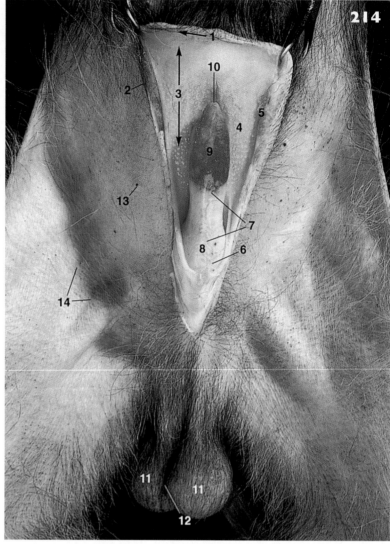

214   Ventral aspect of the inguinal region of a male dog. The prepuce has been opened ventrally to expose the preputial cavity and the glans penis.

1	Preputial orifice (opened ventrally)	8	Bulbus glandis
		9	Pars longa glandis
2	Outer surface } of prepuce	10	External urethral orifice
3	External lamina }	11	Scrotal sacs
4	Lymph nodules	12	Median raphe
5	M. preputialis	13	Teat of undeveloped inguinal
6	Fomix		mammary gland
7	Internal lamina of prepuce	14	Femoral triangle

213   Ventral aspect of the prepuce of a male dog.

1 Preputial orifice
2 Median fold
3 Glans penis within prepuce
4 Caudal extremity of os penis
5 Scrotum

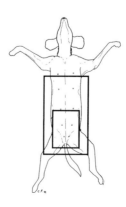

215

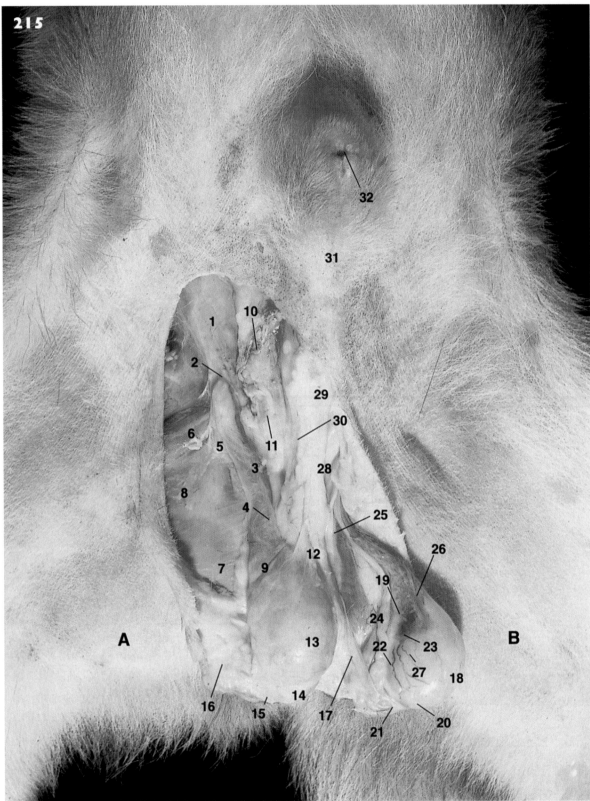

215 Ventral aspect of the inguinal region of a male dog. The scrotal wall has been sectioned on the right side (A) to reveal the testis within the parietal layer of the vaginal tunic. On the left side (B) the parietal layer has been resected to expose the visceral layer of the vaginal tunic covering the testis.

 1 M. obliquus externus abdominis
 2 Superficial inguinal ring
 3 Spermatic cord
 4 Vaginal process
 5 External abdominal fascia
 6 M. pectineus
 7 M. gracilis
 8 M. adductor
 9 M. cremaster within spermatic cord
10 External pudendal artery and vein
11 Superficial inguinal lymph node
12 Spermatic fascia
13 Testis within parietal layer of vaginal tunic
14 Tail of epididymis
15 Scrotal ligament
16 Scrotal wall
17 Median scrotal septum
18 Testis covered in visceral layer of vaginal tunic
19 Ductus deferens
20 Proper ligament of testis
21 Ligament of tail of epididymis
22 Artery and vein of ductus deferens
23 Mesoductus deferens
24 M. cremaster
25 Parietal layer of vaginal tunic
26 Pampiniform plexus of veins
27 Testicular veins
28 Body ⎫
29 Bulbus glandis ⎬ of penis
30 Dorsal artery and vein ⎭
31 Prepuce
32 Preputial orifice

Clinical Note

13 The exposure of the testis on side (A) represents the field seen in the technique of closed castration, i.e. the parietal layer of the vaginal tunic is still intact and the potential space of the peritoneal cavity has not been breached.

18 The exposure of the testis on side (B) represents the field seen in the technique of open castration, i.e. the parietal layer of the vaginal tunic has been incised and thus the potential space of the peritoneal cavity has been breached.

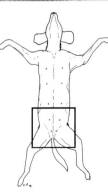

216 Caudal aspect of the perineum of male cat.

1 M. sacrocaudalis ventralis lateralis
2 M. rectococcygeus
3 M. coccygeus
4 M. levator ani
5 M. sphincter ani externus
6 Anus
7 Position of anal sac
8 M. retractor penis overlying M. bulbospongiosum
9 Body of penis
10 M. ischiocavernosus
11 Ischiatic tuberosity
12 Glans penis
13 External urethral orifice
14 Prepuce (opened)
15 Testis covered by parietal layer of vaginal tunic
16 Spermatic cord
17 Sacrotuberous ligament (vestigial)
18 M. obturator internus
19 M. gluteus superficialis
20 M. abductor cruris cranialis (M. coccygeofemoralis)
21 M. biceps femoris
22 M. semitendinosus
23 M. semimembranosus

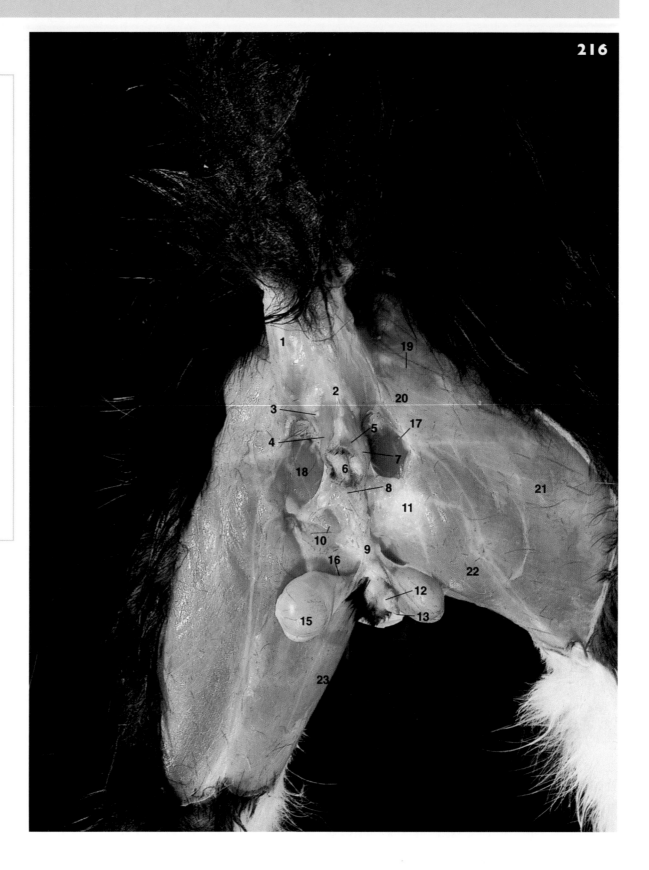

216

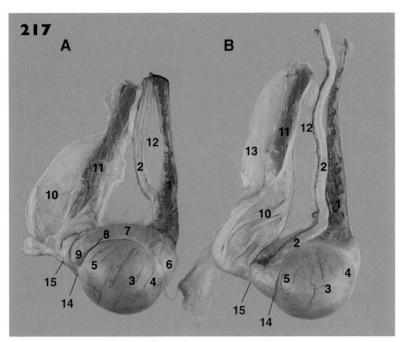

217   Lateral **(A)** and medial **(B)** aspect of the testes of a dog, after removal from the scrotal sacs and severance of the spermatic cords.

1	Pampiniform plexus of veins	10	Parietal layer of vaginal tunic
2	Ductus deferens	11	M. cremaster
3	Testis covered in visceral vaginal tunic	12	Mesofuniculus
		13	External spermatic fascia
4	Head (extremitas capitata)	14	Proper ligament of testis
	} of testis	15	Ligament of tall of epididymis
5	Tail (extremitas caudata)		
6	Head		
7	Body } of epididymis		
8	Sinus		
9	Tail		

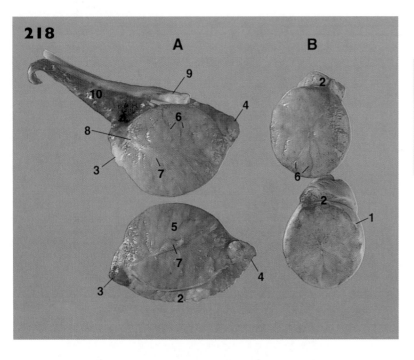

218   Longitudinal **(A)** and transverse **(B)** sections of the testis of a dog.

1	Tunica albuginea (covered in visceral layer of vaginal tunic)	6	Connective tissue septa
		7	Mediastinum testis
2	Body	8	Rete testis
3	Head } of epididymis	9	Ductus deferens
4	Tail	10	Pampiniform plexus of veins
5	Parenchyma testis		

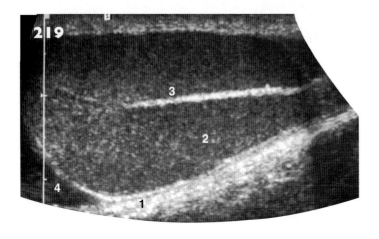

219   **Longitudinal ultrasound scan of the testis of a dog.**

1	Tunics albuginea
2	Parenchyma testis
3	Mediastinum
4	Epididymis

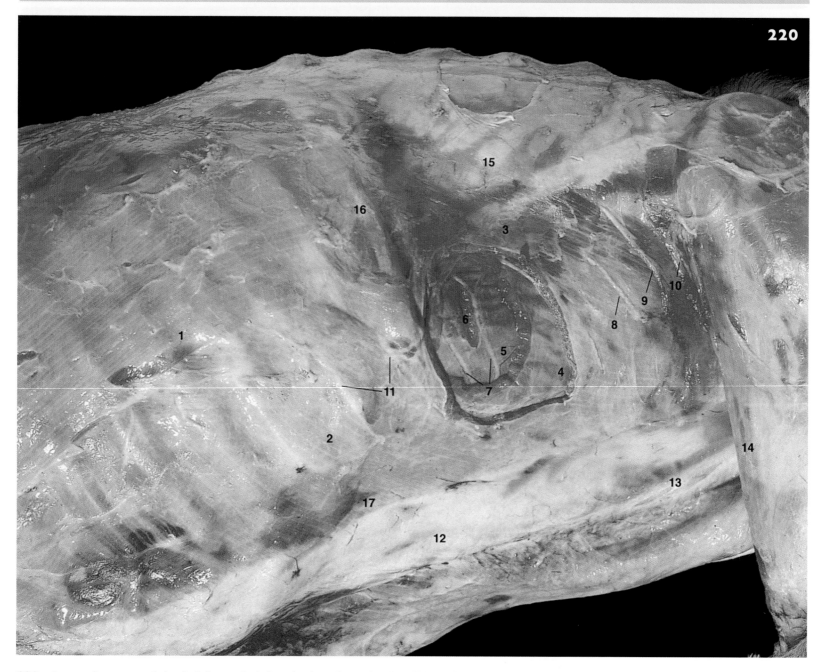

220

220 **Lateral aspect of the left lateral abdominal region of a dog. The skin has been reflected to reveal the muscles of the region, and the abdominal muscle layers have been serially sectioned.**

1 M. latissimus dorsi

2 Pars costalis ⎫ of M. obliquus
3 Pars lumbalis ⎬ externus
            ⎭ abdominis

4 M. obliquus internus abdominis

5 M. transversus abdominis

6 Fascia transversalis

7 Ventral divisions of last thoracic and first lumbar nerves

8 Caudal iliohypogastric nerve (ventral branch of second lumbar nerve)

9 Ilioinguinal nerve (ventral branch of third lumbar nerve)

10 Lateral cutaneous femoral nerve (ventral branch of fourth lumbar nerve)

11 Distal lateral cutaneous branches of intercostal nerves

12 Aponeurosis of M. obliquus externus abdominis

13 M. rectus abdominis (deep to 12)

14 M. sartorius

15 Thoracolumbar fascia

16 Thirteenth (floating) rib

17 Costal arch of costal cartilages

Clinical Note

3, 4 & 5 This dissection of the lateral abdominal wall represents the muscle layers encountered when performing a surgical lateral flank abdominal incision. The level of depth of the incision is judged by assessing the direction of the muscle fibres in each layer of muscle as it is cut through. The level of the muscle transversus abdominis (5) can also be judged by observing the presence of the ventral branches of the spinal nerves (**7**) running over its surface.

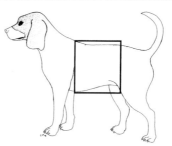

221

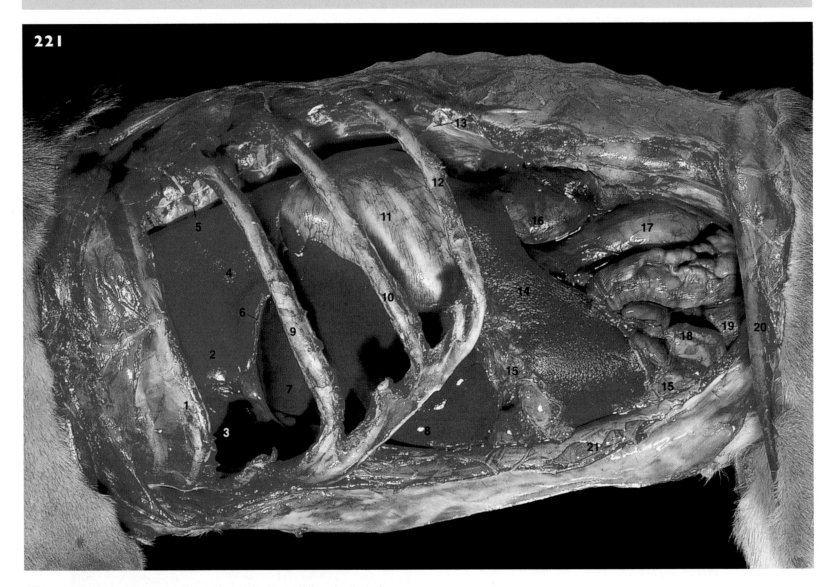

221   Left lateral aspect of the thoracic and abdominal regions of a dog. The thoracic and abdominal lateral walls have been removed, together with the diaphragm, to reveal the topography of the region.

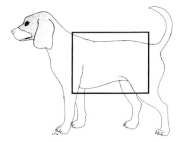

1	Sixth rib	11	Stomach
2	Caudal part of cranial lobe of left lung	12	Twelfth rib
		13	Thirteenth (floating) rib
3	Heart	14	Spleen
4	Caudal lobe of left lung	15	Greater omentum
5	Sympathetic trunk	16	Left kidney
6	Diaphragm (cut)	17	Descending colon
7	Left medial lobe ⎱ of liver	18	Jejunum
8	Left lateral lobe ⎰	19	Urinary bladder
9	Eighth rib	20	M. sartorius
10	Tenth rib	21	M. rectus abdominis

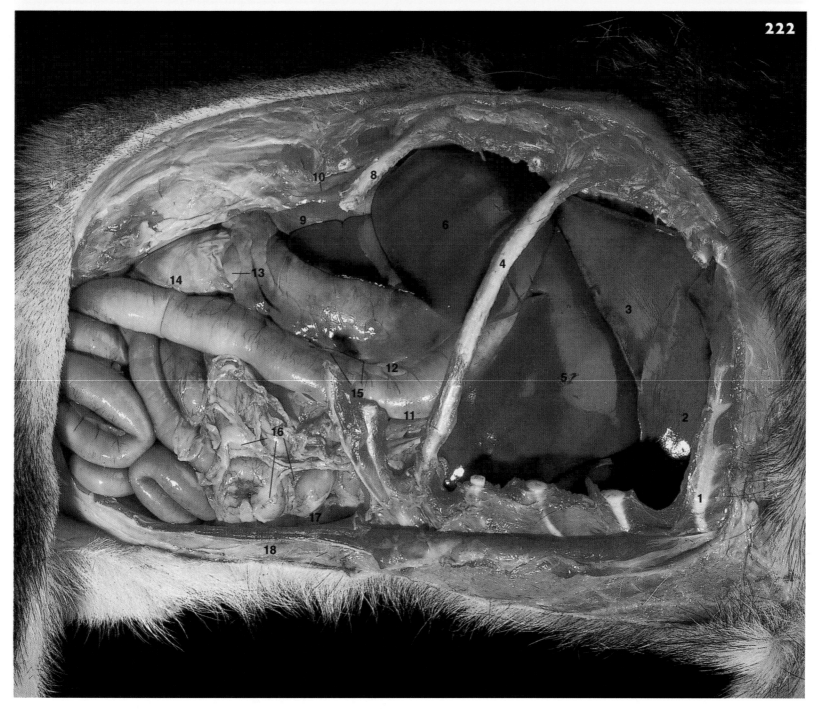

222

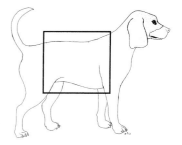

**222   Lateral aspect of the thoracic and abdominal regions of a
dog. The thoracic and abdominal lateral walls have been
removed, together with the diaphragm, to reveal the
topography of the region.**

1	Eighth rib	
2	Middle lobe	of right lung
3	Caudal lobe	
4	Tenth rib	
5	Right medial lobe	of liver
6	Right lateral lobe	(against
7	Caudate lobe	diaphragm)
8	Twelfth rib	
9	Right kidney	
10	Thirteenth (floating) rib	
11	Descending duodenum	
12	Pancreas	
13	Caecum	
14	Descending colon	
15	Mesoduodenum	
16	Greater omentum	
17	Jejunum	
18	M. rectus abdominis	

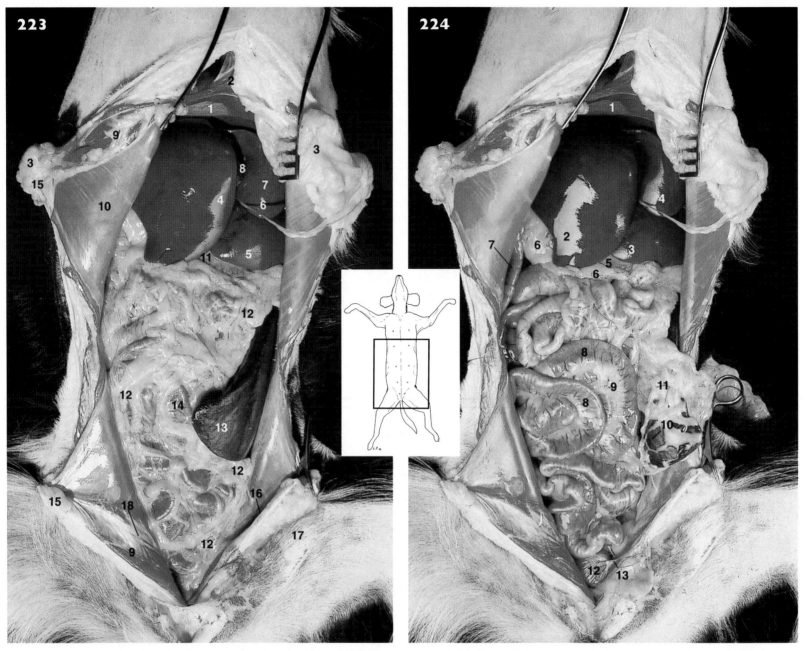

223   Ventral aspect of the opened abdomen of a male dog. The abdominal wall has been sectioned longitudinally in the midline ventrally, along the linea alba, and in a transverse direction at the level of the umbilicus. The greater omentum is seen *in situ*.

1	Diaphragm	10	M. transversus abdominis
2	Xiphoid process of sternum	11	Greater curvature of stomach
3	Falciform ligament	12	Greater omentum
4	Right medial lobe	13	Spleen
5	Left lateral lobe } of liver	14	Jejunum through 12
6	Quadrate lobe	15	Umbilicus
7	Left medial lobe	16	Linea alba
8	Gall bladder	17	Prepuce (reflected)
9	Deep aspect of M. rectus abdominis	18	Caudal deep epigastric artery and vein

224   Ventral aspect of the open abdomen of a male dog. The greater omentum has been reflected cranially to reveal the coils of the intestinal tract.

1	Diaphragm	8	Jejunum
2	Right medial lobe	9	Great mesentery
3	Left lateral lobe } of liver	10	Spleen
4	Left medial lobe	11	Gastrosplenic ligament
5	Greater curvature of stomach	12	Urinary bladder
6	Greater omentum (reflected)	13	Median ligament of the bladder
7	Duodenum		

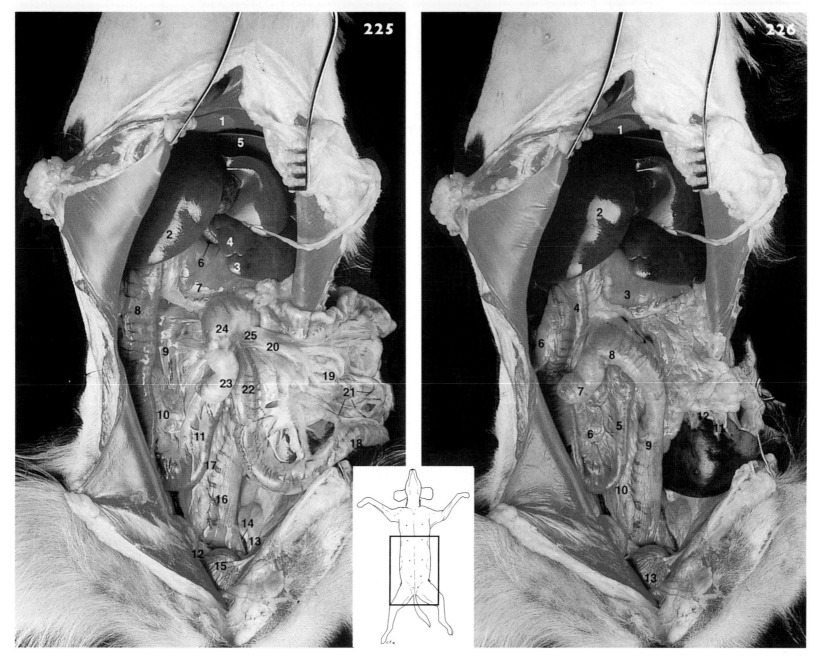

225 Ventral aspect of the open abdomen of a male dog. The greater omentum has been resected from the greater curvature of the stomach, and the coils of the jejunum have been displaced to reveal the ileocolic junction.

226 Ventral aspect of the opened abdomen of a male dog. The intestine has been removed from the level of the ascending duodenum to the ascending colon, and the spleen has been displaced to the left.

1 Diaphragm	15 Urinary bladder
2 Right medial lobe	16 Descending colon
3 Left lateral lobe	17 Mesocolon
4 Quadrate lobe } of liver	18 Jejunum
5 Left medial lobe	19 Great mesentery
6 Lesser curvature } of	20 Mesenteric lymph nodes under fat
7 Greater curvature } stomach	21 Branches of cranial mesenteric arteries and veins
8 Descending duodenum	22 Ileum
9 Mesoduodenum	23 Caecum
10 Right lobe of pancreas	24 Ascending colon
11 Ascending duodenum	25 Root of mesentery
12 Internal inguinal opening	
13 Vaginal process	
14 Testicular vein	

1 Diaphragm	8 Transverse colon
2 Liver	9 Descending colon
3 Parietal surface of stomach	10 Mesocolon
4 Descending duodenum	11 Hilus of spleen
5 Ascending duodenum	12 Gastrosplenic ligament
6 Pancreas in mesoduodenum	13 Urinary bladder
7 Ascending colon	

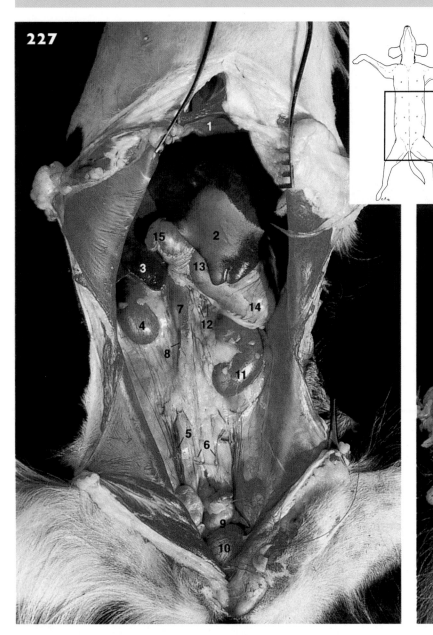

227   **Ventral aspect of the opened abdomen of a male dog. The entire intestinal tract has been removed from the level of the pylorus to the descending colon at the pelvic inlet.**

228   **Ventral aspect of the opened abdomen of a bitch. The gastrointestinal tract has been removed to reveal the urogenital tract *in situ*.**

1 Diaphragm	8 Testicular vein
2 Right medial lobe ⎫	9 Descending colon (transected)
3 Caudate process ⎬ of liver	10 Urinary bladder
of caudate lobe ⎭	11 Left kidney
4 Right kidney	12 Adrenal gland
5 Testicular artery and vein	13 Pylorus ⎫ of stomach
6 Ureters	14 Fundus ⎭
7 Caudal vena cava	15 Duodenum (transected)

1 Liver	9 Vaginal process
2 Caudal pole of right kidney	10 Uterine body
3 Right uterine horn	11 Lateral ligament ⎫ of bladder
4 Right ovary within ovarian	12 Median ligament ⎭
bursa	13 Left uterine horn
5 Suspensory ligament	14 Left ovary within ovarian bursa
6 Mesometrium	15 Mesovarium with ovarian
7 Round ligament of uterus	blood vessels
8 Internal opening of inguinal	16 Left kidney
canal	17 Caudal vena cava

229 Ventral aspect of a section made in the dorsal plane through the thoracic and cranial abdominal region of a dog. The section has been made through the vertebral bodies to demonstrate the topography of the diaphragm and the cranial abdominal organs.

1 Vertebral body	9 Left kidney
2 Crura of diaphragm	10 Renal artery and vein
3 Right caudal lobe of lung	11 Phrenicoabdominal artery and
4 Liver	vein
5 Right kidney	12 Spleen
6 Renal pelvis	13 Stomach
7 Ureter	14 Left caudal lobe of lung
8 Adrenal glands	15 Ribs

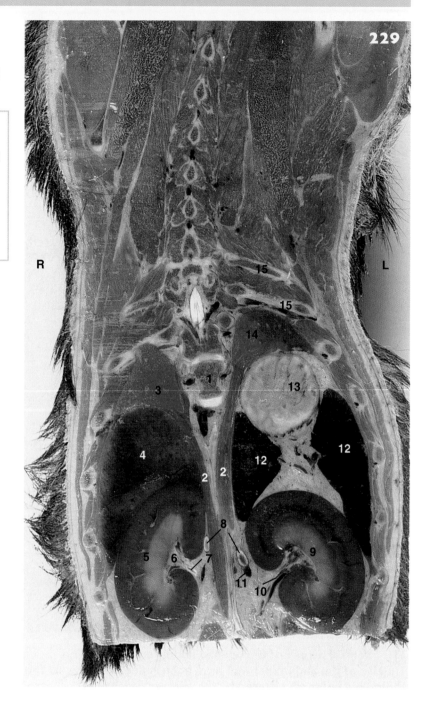

230 Extended field of view ultrasound scan of left flank of a dog to image organs indicated.

1 Liver
2 Spleen
3 Kidney
4 Bowel

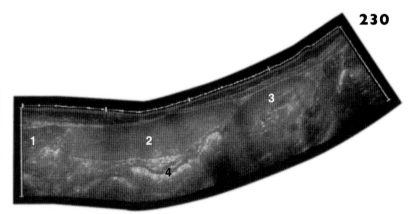

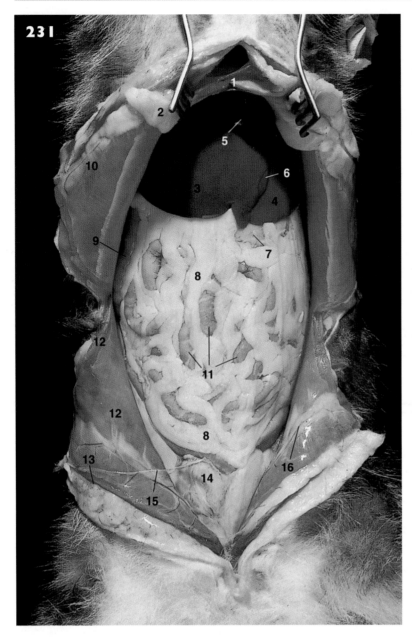

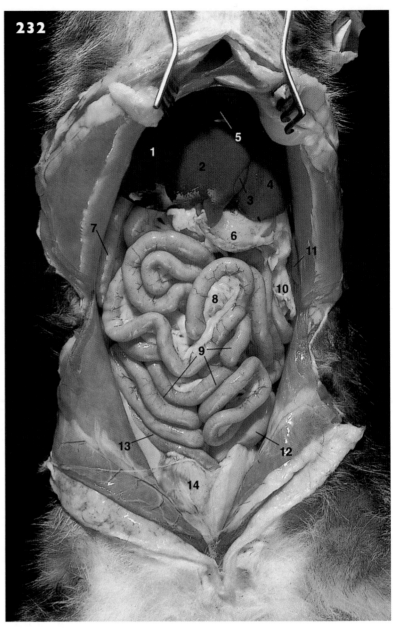

231 Ventral aspect of the opened abdomen of a cat. The muscles of the abdominal wall have been reflected to reveal the abdominal contents covered by the greater omentum.

232 Ventral aspect of the opened abdomen of a cat. The greater omentum has been resected at its attachment to the greater curvature of the stomach.

1 Xiphoid process of sternum	11 Jejunum
2 Fat-laden falciform ligament	12 M. obliquus externus,
3 Right medial lobe ⎫ of liver	M. obliquus internus and
4 Left lateral lobe ⎭	M. transversus abdominis
5 Gall bladder	13 M. rectus abdominis
6 Quadrate lobe of liver	14 Urinary bladder
7 Stomach	15 Median ligament of bladder
8 Greater omentum	16 Deep caudal epigastric vessels
9 Descending duodenum	
10 Parietal peritoneum overlying	
deep rectal sheath	

1 Right lateral lobe ⎫	8 Great mesentery
2 Right medial lobe ⎬ of liver	9 Jejunum
3 Quadrate lobe ⎪	10 Gastrosplenic ligament
4 Left lateral lobe ⎭	11 Spleen
5 Gall bladder	12 Descending colon
6 Greater curvature of stomach	13 Right uterine horn
7 Descending duodenum	14 Urinary bladder

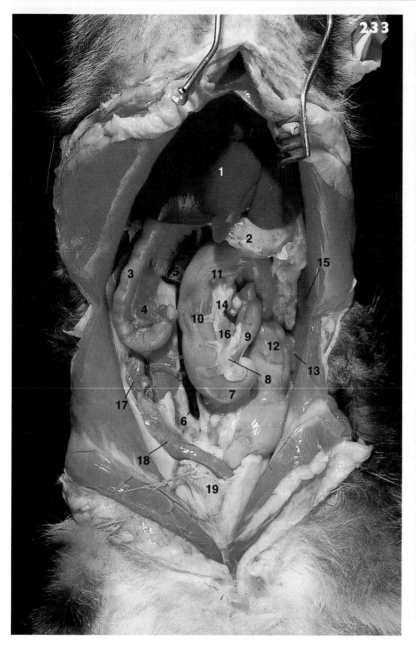

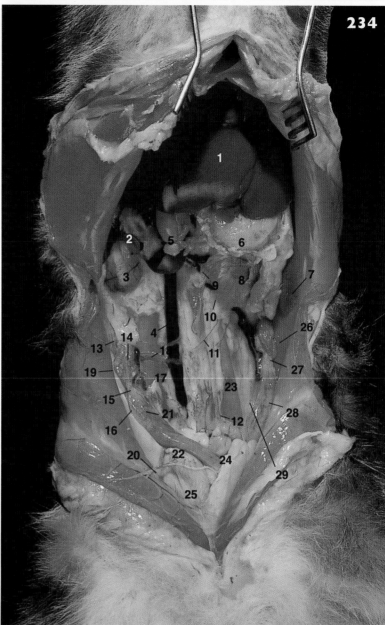

233 Ventral aspect of the opened abdomen of a female cat. The small intestine has been resected at the level of the descending duodenum and the terminal portion of the ileum.

234 Ventral aspect of the opened abdomen of a female cat. The intestinal tract has been removed to reveal the urogenital tract *in situ*.

1	Liver	10	Ascending colon
2	Stomach	11	Transverse colon
3	Duodenum	12	Descending colon
4	Right lobe of pancreas (in mesoduodenum)	13	Left ovary
		14	Root of mesentery
5	Caudate lobe of liver	15	Spleen
6	Caudal vena cava	16	Mesenteric lymph nodes
7	Ceacum	17	Right ovary
8	Ileocolic junction	18	Right uterine horn
9	Ileum	19	Urinary bladder

1	Liver	16	Proper ligament of ovary
2	Caudate lobe of 1	17	Mesovarium
3	Right kidney	18	Ovarian artery and vein
4	Caudal vena cava	19	Uterine tube
5	Duodenum (cut)	20	Round ligament running to internal inguinal ring
6	Stomach	
7	Spleen	21	Uterine branch of 18
8	Left kidney	22	Right uterine horn
9	Renal vein	23	M. psoas
10	Ovarian vessel	24	Descending colon (cut)
11	Aorta	25	Urinary bladder
12	Ureter	26	Lateral aspect of left ovary
13	Suspensory ligament	or right	27	Uterine tube
14	Medial aspect	ovary	28	Left uterine horn
15	Entrance to ovarian bursa	29	Mesometrium

Clinical Note

7 Note that the feline caecum is not coiled upon itself as is found in the dog (Fig. 225, **23**).

235

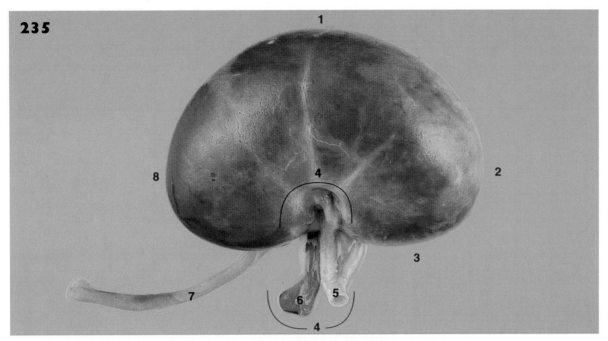

235   Dorsal aspect of the kidney of a dog.

1 Convex lateral border
2 Cranial pole
3 Medial border
4 Hilus
5 Renal artery
6 Renal vein
7 Ureter
8 Caudal pole

236

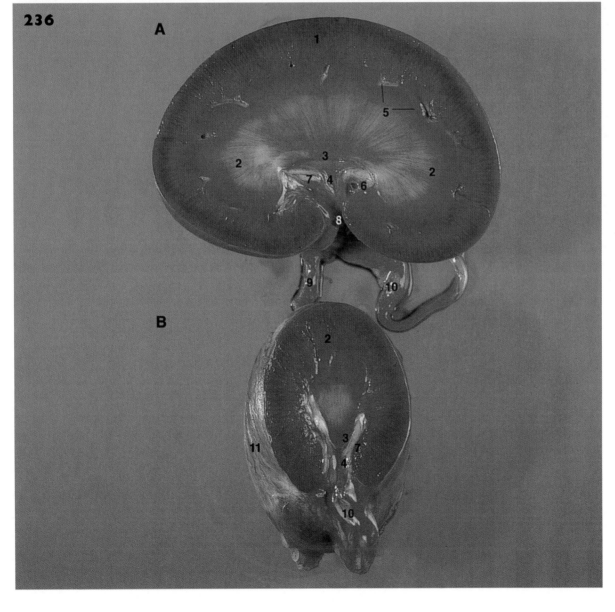

236   Dorsal aspect of a midfrontal section (A) and cross section (B) of the kidney of a dog.

1 Cortex with medullary rays
2 Medulla
3 Crest
4 Renal pelvis
5 Interlobar arteries and veins breaking up to form arcuate vessels
6 Sinus
7 Fat
8 Hilus
9 Renal artery
10 Ureter
11 Renal capsule

237   Frontal section in the dorsal plane of the kidney of a dog.

I	Cortex
2	Pyramid
3	Medulla
4	Fat (in sinus)
5	Interlobar vessels
6	Arcuate vessels

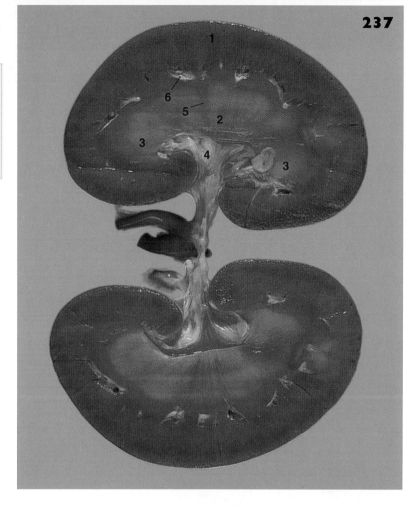

237

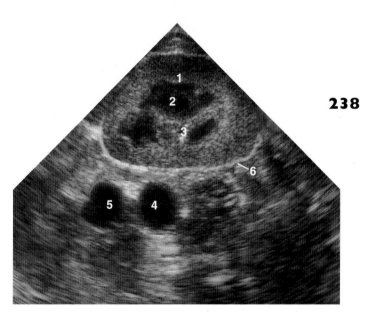

238

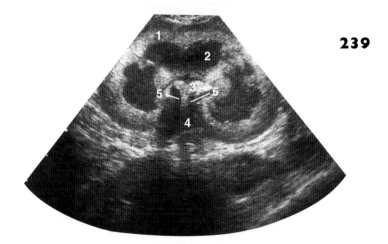

239

238   Transverse ultrasound scan of the kidney of a dog, illustrating the contrast between the echogenicity of the cortex and that of the medulla.

I	Renal cortex	4	Aorta
2	Renal medulla	5	Vena cava
3	Renal pelvis	6	Renal capsule

239   Ultrasound scan of the kidney of a dog, made in the dorsal plane, illustrating the contrast between the echogenicity of the cortex and that of the medulla. The renal pelvis produces strong echoes and appears white at the centre of the kidney outline.

I	Renal cortex
2	Renal medulla
3	Renal pelvis
4	Hilus
5	Renal vessels

Clinical Note
This scan is in a plane similar to that in the gross anatomical sectioned kidney.

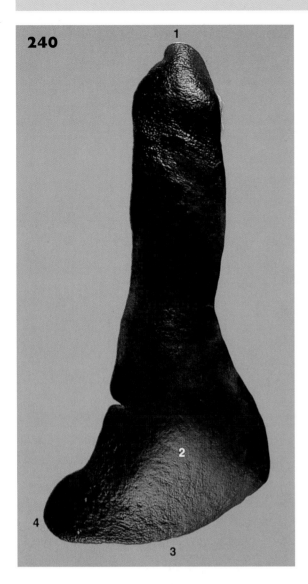

240

240   Parietal surface of the spleen of a dog.

1 Dorsal extremity
2 Parietal surface
3 Ventral extremity
4 Cranially directed tip

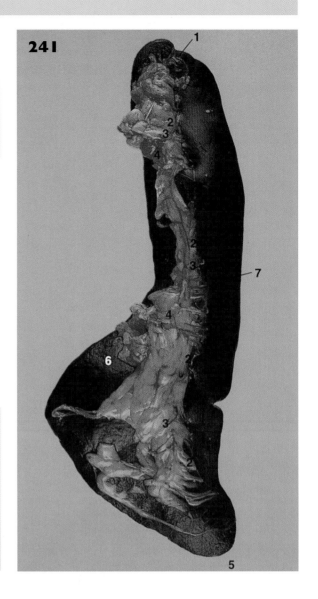

241

241   Visceral surface of the spleen of a dog.

1 Dorsal extremity
2 Hilus
3 Attachment of gastrosplenic ligament
4 Branches of splenic artery and vein
5 Ventral extremity
6 Intestinal surface
7 Gastric surface

242

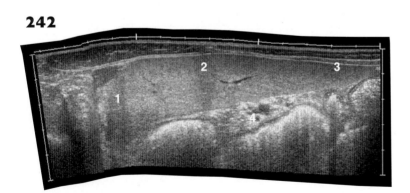

242   Extended field of view ultrasound scan of left flank of a dog to image entire spleen.

1 Dorsal extremity   3 Ventral extremity
2 Body of spleen   4 Bowel

243   Ultrasound scan of the spleen of a dog, showing the splenic vessels running through the splenic tissue.

1	Spleen
2	Splenic vessels

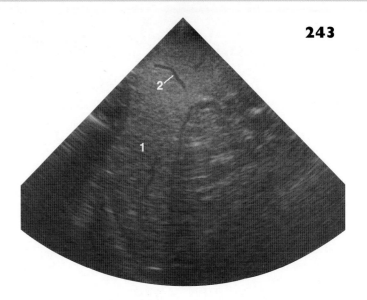

243

244   Ultrasound scan of the kidney and spleen of a dog, illustrating the contrast in echogenicity between these organs. On the left, the spleen can be seen to abutt onto the kidney.

1	Spleen
2	Renal cortex
3	Renal medulla

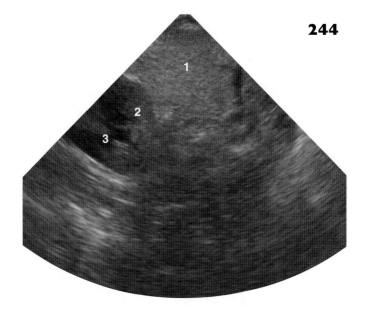

244

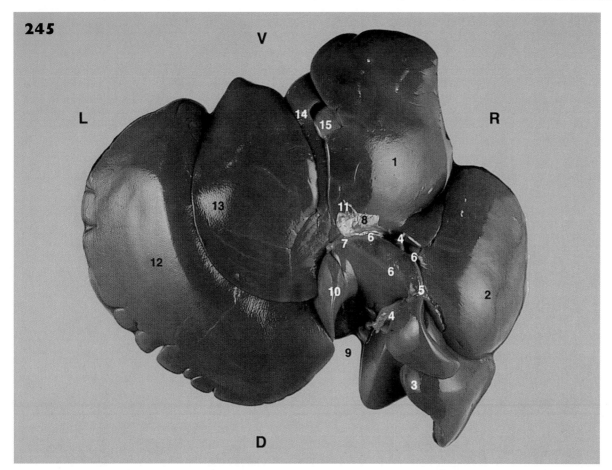

245 **Diaphragmatic surface of the liver of a dog. Orientation ventrally (V), dorsally (D), left (L) and right (R) is indicated.**

1 Right medial lobe
2 Right lateral lobe
3 Caudate lobe
4 Caudal vena cava
5 Right triangular ligament
6 Coronary ligament
7 Left triangular ligament
8 Fragment of diaphragm
9 Oesophageal notch
10 Papillary process of caudate lobe
11 Falciform ligament
12 Left lateral lobe
13 Left medial lobe
14 Quadrate lobe
15 Gall bladder

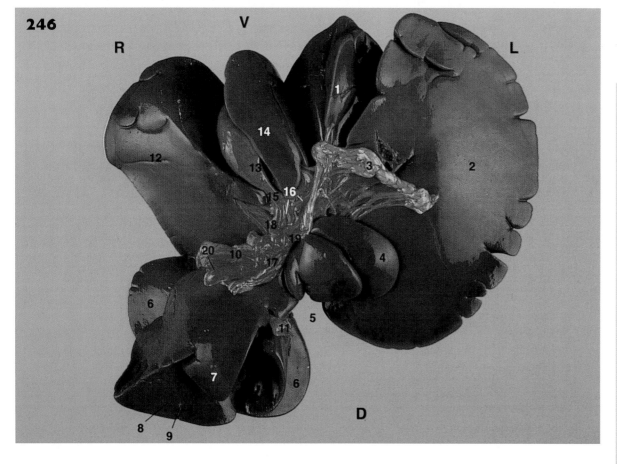

246 **Visceral surface of the liver of a dog. Orientation ventrally (V), dorsally (D), left (L) and right (R) is indicated.**

1 Left medial lobe
2 Left lateral lobe
3 Lesser omentum (hepatogastric ligament)
4 Papillary process of caudate lobe
5 Oesophageal notch
6 Right lateral lobe
7 Caudate process of caudate lobe
8 Renal fossa
9 Hepatorenal ligament
10 Lesser omentum (hepatoduodenal ligament)
11 Caudal vena cava
12 Right medial lobe
13 Gall bladder
14 Quadrate lobe
15 Cystic duct
16 Hepatic ducts
17 Bile duct
18 Portal vein
19 Hepatic artery
20 Gastroduodenal artery

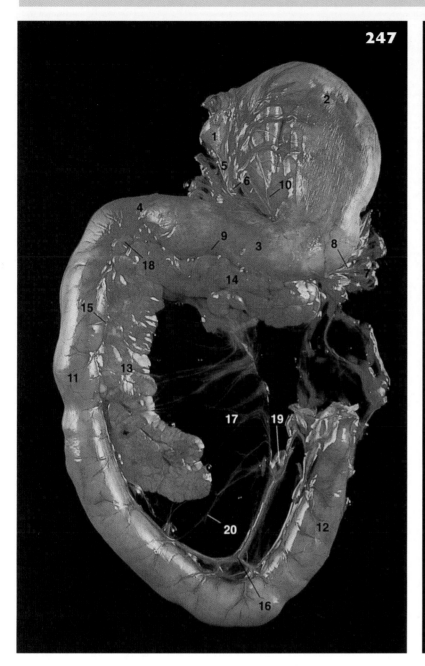

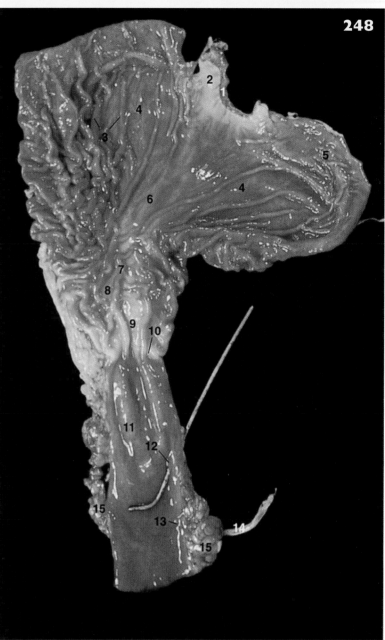

247   Ventral aspect of the stomach, duodenum and pancreas of a dog.

248   Opened stomach of a dog. The organ has been cut along its greater curvature to reveal the mucosal lining. The probe occupies the point of entry of the major duodenal papilla.

1	Cardia	13	Right lobe ⎫ of pancreas
2	Fundus	14	Left lobe ⎭
3	Pyloric antrum	15	Cranial pancreaticoduodenal
4	Pylorus		artery (from coeliac artery)
5	Lesser omentum	16	Caudal pancreaticoduodenal
6	Left gastric artery		artery (from cranial
7	Greater omentum		mesenteric artery)
8	Left gastroepiploic artery	17	Mesoduodenum
9	Right gastroepiploic artery	18	Duodenal lymph node
10	Lymphatic vessels	19	Mesenteric lymph node
11	Descending duodenum	20	Gastroduodenal branches of
12	Ascending duodenum		autonomic nerve fibres

1	Cardia	9	Pyloric canal
2	Region of cardiac glands	10	Pylorus
3	Gastric folds	11	Duodenum
4	Region of gastric glands	12	Major duodenal papilla (with
	(proper)		probe)
5	Fundus	13	Minor duodenal papilla
6	Body	14	Pancreatic duct
7	Region of pyloric glands	15	Pancreatic tissue
8	Pyloric antrum		

249

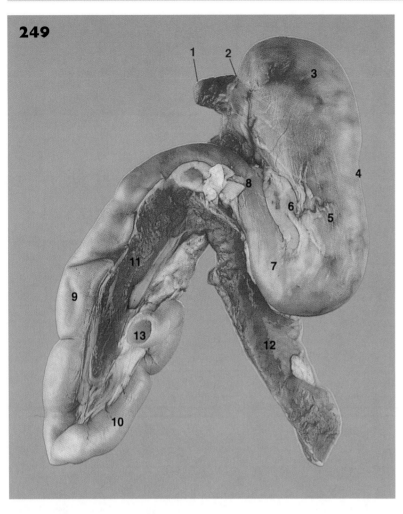

250   Ileocolic orifice of a dog. The ileum and the ascending colon have been opened to reveal the change in the nature of the mucosal lining.

1	Ileum
2	Caecum
3	Caecal fold
4	Ileocolic orifice and sphincter
5	Accessory ileocaecal fold
6	Caecocolic orifice
7	Ascending colon
8	Lymph follicles

250

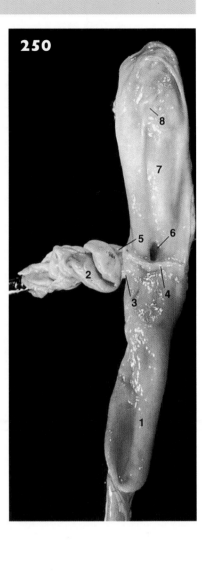

249   Stomach, duodenum and pancreas of a cat.

1	Oesophagus	8	Pylorus
2	Cardia	9	Descending duodenum
3	Fundus	10	Ascending duodenum
4	Greater curvature	11	Right lobe
5	Body	12	Left lobe
6	Lesser curvature	13	Jejunum
7	Pyloric antrum		

4 Greater curvature, 5 Body, 6 Lesser curvature } of stomach

11 Right lobe, 12 Left lobe } of pancreas

**251   Intestinal tract of a cat.
The viscera have been
removed from the abdomen
and arranged to display the
ileocolic junction and the
simple, uncoiled blind sac of
the caecum of a cat.**

1 Coils of jejunum
2 Great mesentery
3 Mesenteric lymph nodes
4 Mesenteric arteries and veins
5 Ileum
6 Caecum
7 Ascending colon
8 Transverse colon
9 Descending colon

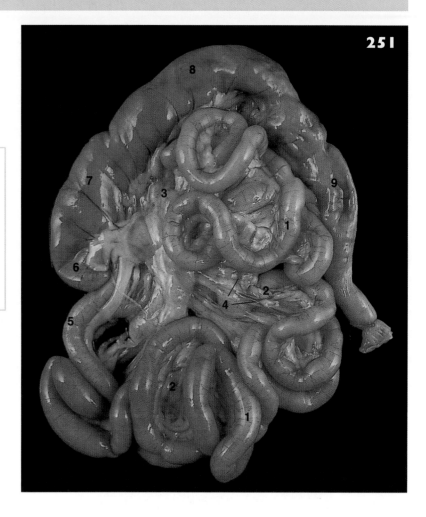

**252   Kidney, spleen and liver
of a cat.**

1	Kidney with capsular veins
2	Renal hilus
3	Parietal surface
4	Dorsal border } of spleen
5	Cranial border
6	Visceral surface
7	Left lateral lobe
8	Left medial lobe
9	Quadrate lobe } of liver
10	Right medial lobe
11	Right lateral lobe
12	Caudate lobe
13	Caudate process } of 12
14	Papillary process
15	Porta
16	Gall bladder
17	Dorsal border of liver

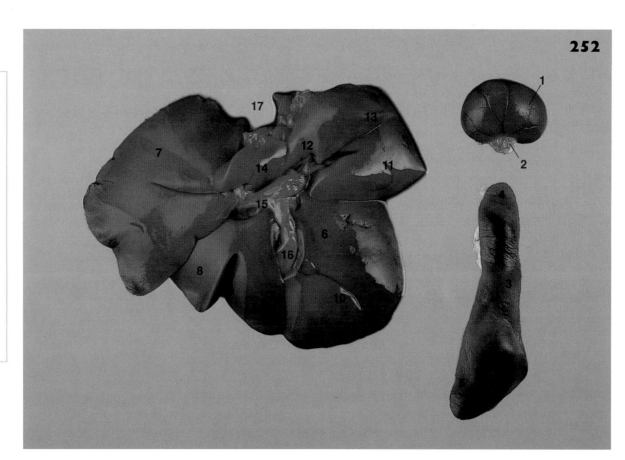

253

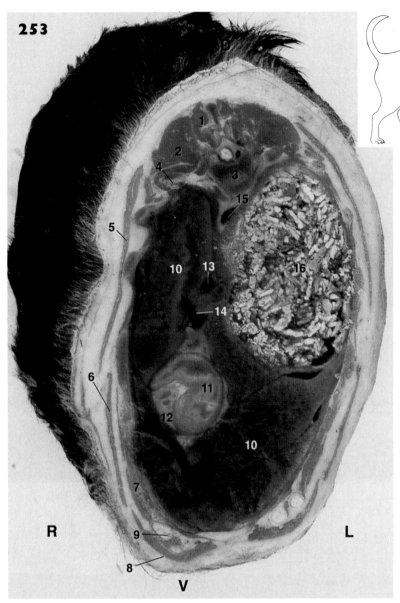

254

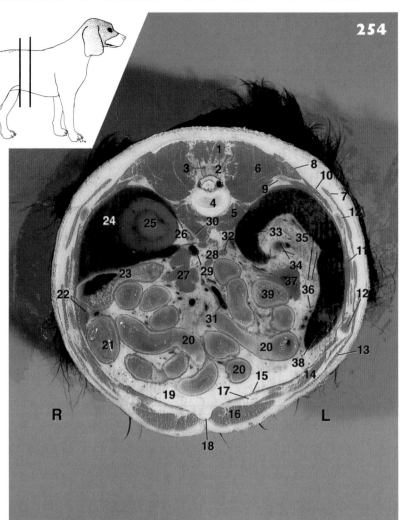

253   Cranial aspect of a transverse section through the abdomen of a dog, at the level of the eleventh thoracic vertebra. Dorsal (D), ventral (V), left (L) and right (R) orientations are indicated.

1	Mm. multifidus thoracis and lumborum	8	M. rectus abdominis
2	Mm. longissimus thoracis and lumborum	9	Costal cartilages
		10	Liver
3	Eleventh thoracic vertebra	11	Pylorus
4	Rib	12	Pancreas
5	M. latissimus dorsi	13	Caudal vena cava
6	M. obliquus externus abdominis	14	Portal vein
		15	Aorta
7	M. intercostalis	16	Body of stomach (with contents)

254   Cranial face of a transverse section through the abdominal region of a dog, at the level of the first and second lumbar vertebrae. Left (L) and right (R) orientations are indicated.

1	Mm. multifidus thoracis and lumborum	19	Greater omentum
2	Second lumbar vertebra	20	Jejunum
3	First lumbar vertebra	21	Descending duodenum
4	Invertebral disc	22	Pancreas
5	M. psoas major	23	Transverse colon
6	Mm. longissimus thoracis and lumborum	24	Caudate lobe of liver
		25	Right kidney
7	M. latissimus dorsi	26	Renal hilus
8	M. iliocostalis	27	Mesenteric lymph nodes
9	Thirteenth (floating) rib	28	Root of mesentery
10	M. serratus dorsalis	29	Caudal vena cava
11	M. intercostalis	30	Aorta
12	Twelfth rib and costochondral junction	31	Cranial mesenteric vein
		32	Lumbar lymph nodes
13	M. obliquus externus abdominis	33	Dorsal extremity of spleen
14	M. obliquus internus abdominis	34	Cranial pole of left kidney
15	M. transversus abdominis	35	Gastrosplenic ligament
16	M. rectus abdominis	36	Splenic vessels
17	Eleventh costal cartilage	37	Pancreas
18	Linea alba	38	Caudal extremity of spleen
		39	Descending colon

255 Cranial aspect of a transverse section through the abdomen of a dog at the level of the second lumbar vertebra.

1	Second lumbar vertebra	10	Spleen
2	Right kidney	11	Ascending duodenum
3	Caudate lobe of liver	12	Root of mesentery
4	Descending duodenum	13	M. transversus abdominis
5	Ascending colon	14	M. rectus abdominis
6	Pancreas	15	M. obliquus abdominis externus
7	Jejunum	16	M. obliquus abdominis internus
8	Left kidney	17	Linea alba
9	Descending colon	18	Adrenal gland

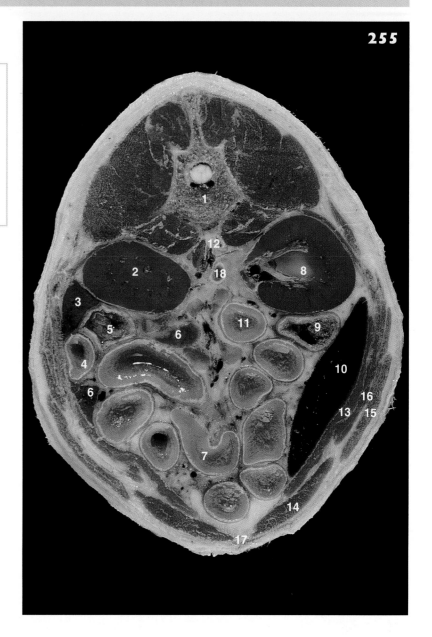

255

256

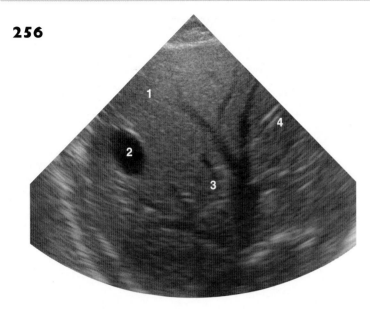

256   Transverse ultrasound scan of the liver of a dog. The gall bladder is seen as a black circular image.

1 Liver	3 Hepatic veins
2 Gall bladder	4 Portal veins

Clinical Note
4   Portal veins have walls that give strong echoes, and appear as black structures with bright walls.

257

257   Longitudinal ultrasound scan of the liver of a dog. The heart can be seen through the diaphragm at depth.

1 Gall bladder	4 Hepatic vein
2 Diaphragm	5 Stomach
3 Heart	

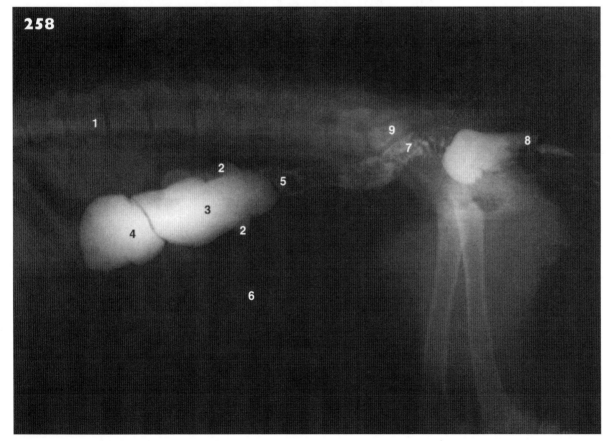

258

258   Lateral radiograph of the abdomen of a dog. A barium enema has been administered to demonstrate the location of the large intestine.

1	First lumbar vertebra
2	Caecum
3	Ascending colon
4	Transverse colon
5	Descending colon
6	Jejunum
7	Rectum
8	Anus
9	Sacrum

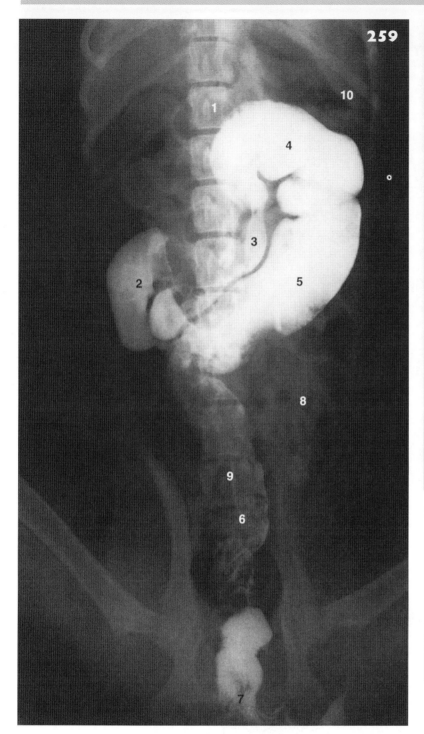

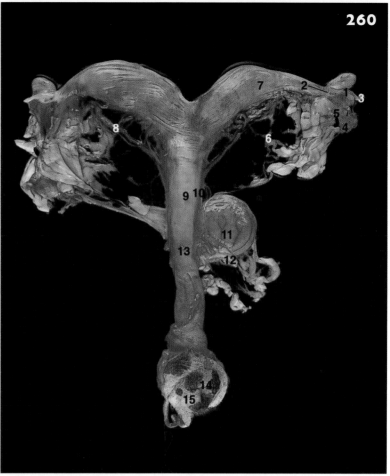

260 Dorsal aspect of the genital tract of a bitch.

1	Ovarian bursa	9	Uterine body
2	Opening of ovarian bursa	10	Uterine artery
3	Suspensory ligament of ovary	11	Urinary bladder
4	Ovarian artery	12	Ureter
5	Mesovarium	13	Vagina
6	Mesometrium	14	Vulva
7	Uterine horn	15	Labia
8	Uterine branch of 4		

259 Ventrodorsal radiograph of the abdomen of a dog. A barium enema has been administered to demonstrate the location of the large intestine.

1	Thirteenth thoracic vertebra	6	Rectum
2	Caecum	7	Anus
3	Ascending colon	8	Jejunum
4	Transverse colon	9	Seventh lumbar vertebra
5	Descending colon	10	Spleen

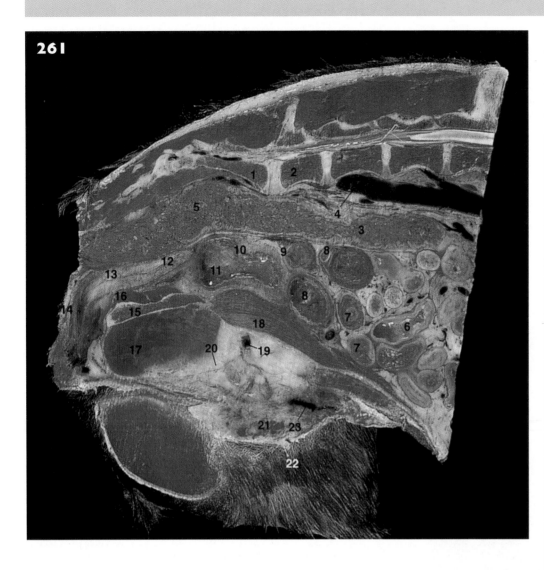

261

1   Sacrum
2   Seventh lumbar vertebra
3   Descending colon
4   Caudal vena cava
5   Rectum
6   Jejunum
7   Duodenum
8   Uterine horn
9   Uterine body
10   Cervix
11   Urinary bladder
12   Vagina
13   Vestibule
14   Vulva
15   Pubis
16   M. obturatorius internus
17   M. adductor
18   M. rectus abdominis
19   External pudendal artery
     and vein
20   Superficial inguinal lymph
     node
21   Inguinal mammary gland
22   Teat
23   Caudal superficial epigastric
     artery and vein

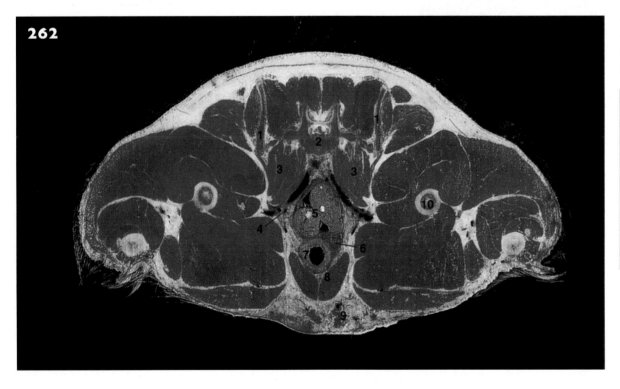

262

262   Cranial aspect of a
transverse section of the
trunk of a bitch, at the level of
the seventh lumbar vertebra.

1   Wing of ilium
2   Seventh lumbar vertebra
3   M. iliopsoas
4   Internal iliac artery and vein
5   Rectum
6   Uterine body
7   Urinary bladder
8   M. rectus abdominis
9   Mammary gland
10   Femur

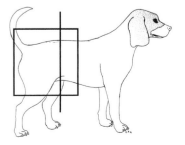

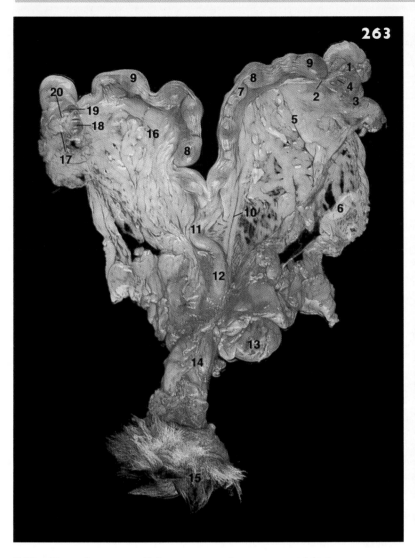

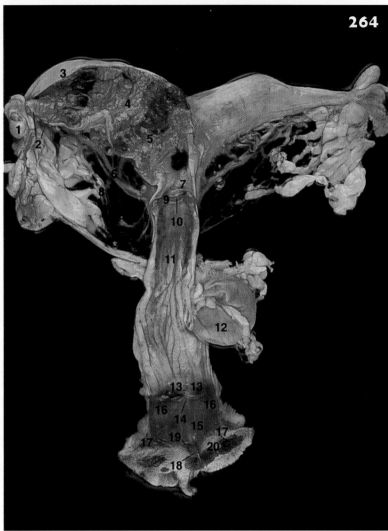

263   Dorsal aspect of the uterus of a pregnant bitch.

1	Suspensory ligament } of	11	Uterine body
2	Proper ligament } ovary	12	Vagina
3	Mesovarium	13	Urinary bladder
4	Opening of ovarian bursa	14	Vestibule
5	Mesometrium (broad	15	Vulva
	ligament)	16	Uterine branch of ovarian
6	Round ligament		artery and vein
7	Uterine horn	17	Ovarian bursa (opened)
8	Loci of conceptuses	18	Ovary bearing corpora lutea
9	Area of zonary band	19	Infundibulum
10	Uterine artery and vein	20	Oviduct

264   Dorsal aspect of the genital tract of a bitch. The tract, which has been opened dorsally, illustrates an endometrial lining that is typical of a postpaturient bitch.

1	Ovary extruded from bursa	10	External uterine orifice
2	Uterine tube	11	Vagina
3	Uterine horn	12	Urinary bladder
4	Endometrium	13	Mucosal folds
5	Area of detached placentation	14	External urethral orifice
	(zonary)	15	Vestibule
6	Uterine branch of ovarian	16	Vestibule bulb
	artery and vein	17	M. constrictor vestibuli
7	Uterine body	18	Clitoris
8	Mesometrium (broad ligament)	19	Fossa clitoridis
9	Cervix	20	Labia

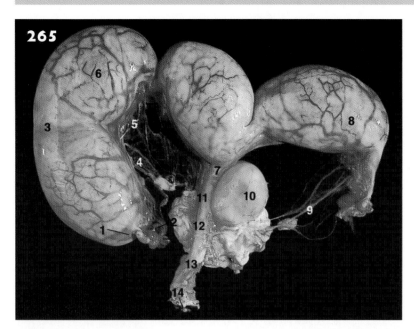

265 **Dorsal aspect of the uterus of a pregnant cat, showing the location of four conceptuses.**

1	Ovary with corpora lutea	7	Uterine body
2	Mesovarium with ovarian artery and vein	8	Right uterine horn
3	Gravid left uterine horn	9	Round ligament
4	Mesometrium	10	Urinary bladder
5	Uterine branch of ovarian artery	11	Level of cervix
6	Placental bands seen through myometrium	12	Vagina
		13	Vestibule
		14	Vulva

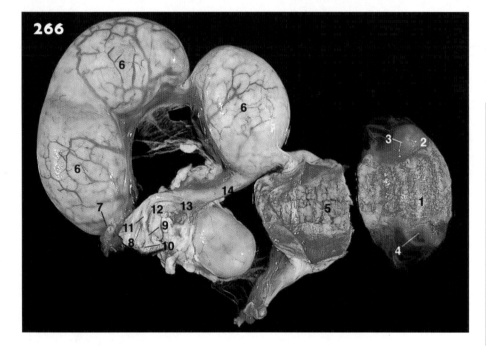

266 **Dorsal aspect of the uterus of a pregnant cat. The loculus of the right horn has been opened and the foetus, surrounded by the foetal membranes and zonary placenta, has been displaced. The vulva, vestibule and vagina have been opened dorsally.**

1 Zonary placental band surrounding foetus
2 Foetus within foetal membranes
3 Cranium
4 Tall and pelvic limb of foetus
5 Myometrium (stripped of endometrium)
6 Intact loculi
7 Ovary with corpora lutea
8 Vulva
9 Vestibule
10 Fossa clitoridis enclosing clitoris
11 External urethral orifice
12 Vagina
13 Cervix
14 Uterine body

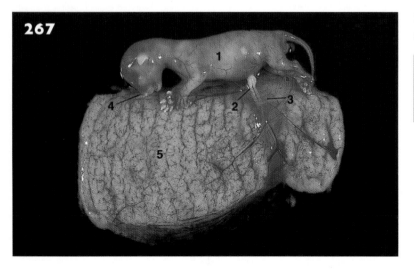

267 **Feline foetus with opened foetal membranes and sectioned placental band.**

1	Foetus	4	Opened foetal membranes
2	Umbilicus	5	Placental band
3	Umbilical vessels		

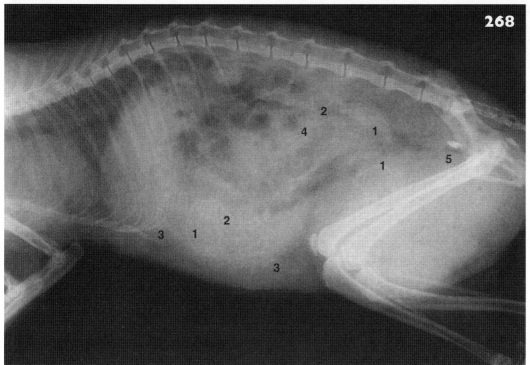

268   Lateral radiograph of the abdomen of a pregnant cat.

1 Foetal skulls
2 Foetal vertebrae
3 Foetal limbs
4 Foetal ribs
5 Pelvic inlet

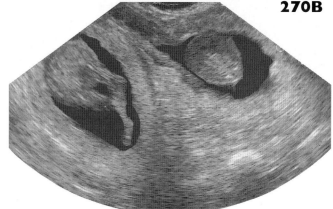

270A

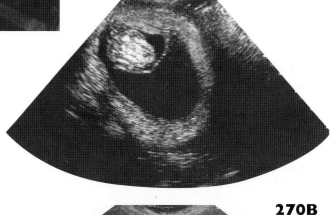

270B

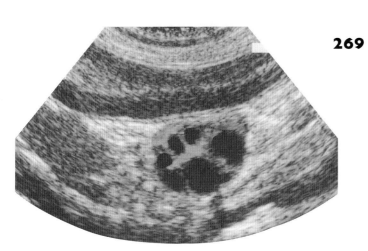

269

269   Ultrasound scan of the ovary of a bitch, made through the lateral abdominal wall. The muscle layers can be seen at the top of the scan and the ovary occupies the centre of the field. The darkened circular areas on the ovarian surface are follicles.

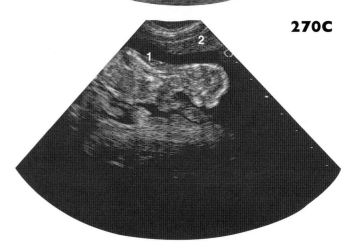

270C

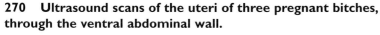

270   Ultrasound scans of the uteri of three pregnant bitches, through the ventral abdominal wall.

A   Early pregnancy, showing the conceptus surrounded by the placental membranes. The lumen of the uterus appears black (anechoic).

B   Twin pregnancy showing conceptuses lying within the lumen of the uterine horns. The foetuses are enlarged in cross section.

C   Scan of the thoracic region of a foetus in late pregnancy. The foetal ribs are evident as strong, white echoes lying in the centre of the field and extending to the left (1). The placentary band can be seen peripheral to this (2).

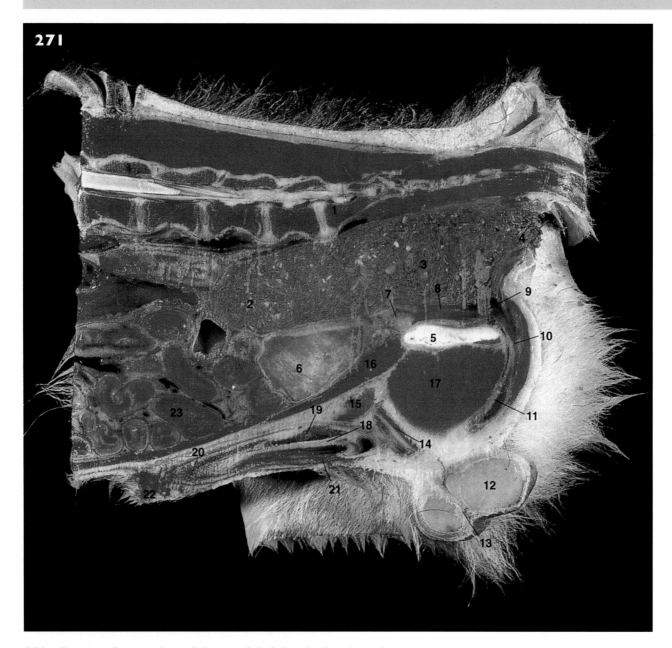

271   Paramedian section of the caudal abdominal and pelvic cavities of a male dog, showing the topography of the pelvic contents and the external genitalia.

1	Sacrum	13	Scrotum
2	Descending colon	14	Spermatic cord
3	Rectum	15	Superficial inguinal lymph node
4	Anus	16	M. rectus abdominis
5	Pubis	17	M. adductor
6	Urinary bladder	18	Os penis
7	Prostate	19	Bulbus glandis
8	Pelvic urethra	20	Pars longa glandis
9	Penile urethra	21	Penile urethra in ventral groove
10	M. ischiocavernosus	22	Prepuce
11	Corpus cavernosum penis	23	Jejunum
12	Testis		

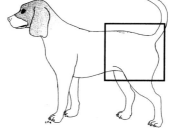

272   Cranial aspect of transverse sections through the seventh lumbar (A) and first caudal (B) vertebrae of a male dog, showing the topography of the pelvic contents.

1   Ilium
2   Seventh lumbar vertebra
3   Intervertebral disc
4   Annulus fibrosus
5   Nucleus pulposus
6   Rectum
7   Urinary bladder
8   M. transversus abdominis
9   M. obliquus internus abdominis
10 M. obliquus externus abdominis
11 M. rectus abdominis
12 M. protractor preputii
13 Linea alba
14 Prepuce
15 Preputial branches of external pudendal artery
16 Mm. iliocostalis and longissimus lumborum
17 Mm. iliacus and psoas major
18 Hypogastric lymph node
19 M. tensor fasciae latae
20 First caudal vertebra
21 Prostate gland
22 Pelvic urethra
23 Bulbus glandis of penis
24 Os penis
25 Penile urethra
26 Superficial branch of dorsal artery of penis
27 M. coccygeus
28 Gluteal muscle mass

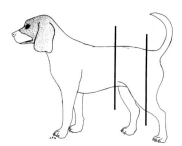

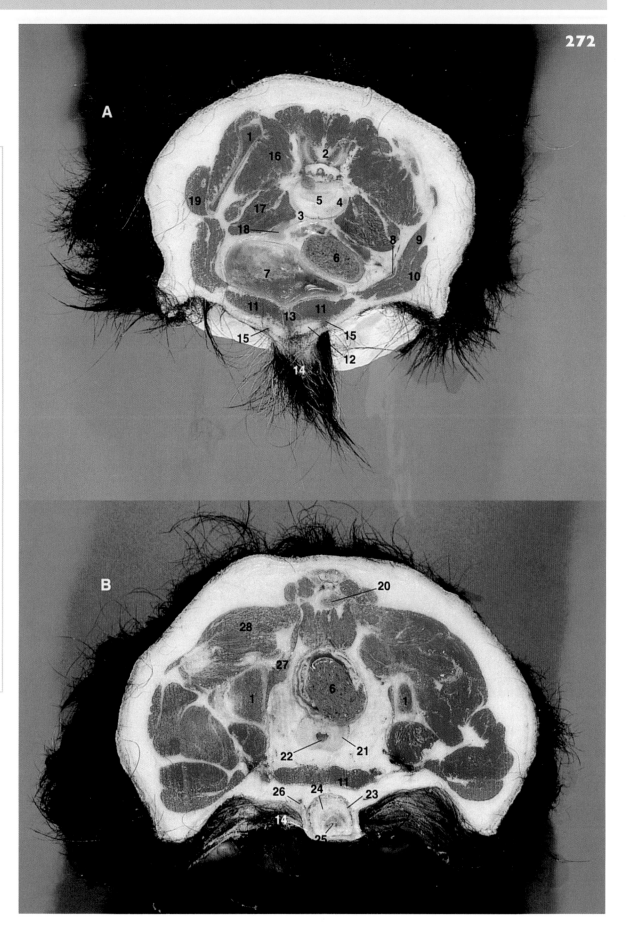

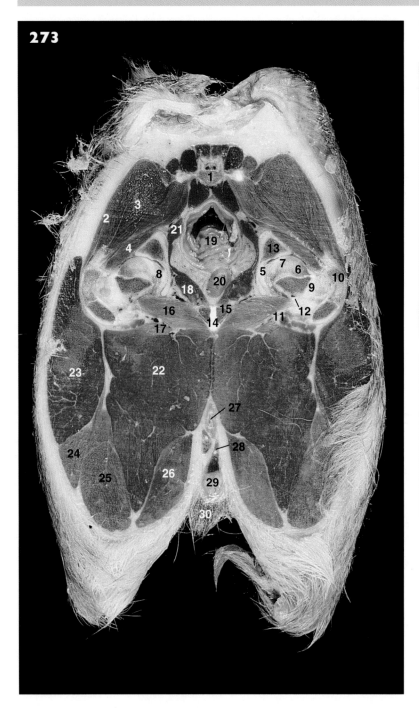

273

1	Third caudal vertebra	15	Pubis
2	M. gluteus superficialis	16	M. obturator externus
3	M. gluteus medius	17	M. quadratus femoris
4	M. gluteus profundus	18	M. pubocaudalis
5	Acetabulum	19	Rectum
6	Femoral head	20	Pelvic urethra
7	Articular surface of 6	21	M. levator ani
8	Ligament of the head of the femur (Teres ligament, round ligament)	22	M. adductor
		23	M. biceps femoris
		24	M. semitendinosus
9	Femoral neck	25	M. semimembranosus
10	Greater trochanter	26	M. gracilis
11	Lesser trochanter	27	Penis
12	Trochanteric fossa	28	Spermatic cord
13	Body of ilium	29	Testis
14	Pelvic symphysis	30	Scrotum

Clinical Note

21   This muscle in combination with the coccygeus muscle form the structure of the pelvic diaphragm which lies to either side of the rectum offering lateral support during the contractions of defaecation. In older dogs, particularly males, this support may degenerate as these muscles atrophy. This causes the rectum to deviate to the side of breakdown during attempted defaecation with a resulting swelling developing subcutaneously, lateral to the anus in the perineal region. This is the clinical condition referred to as perineal hernia.

274 Ultrasound scan through the ventral abdominal wall of a male dog, made in the prepubic location. The urinary bladder can be seen with the prostate immediately adjacent to it.

1 Urinary bladder
2 Prostate gland

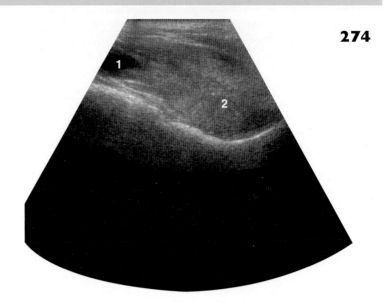

274

275 Caudal ultrasound scan through the ventral abdominal wall of a male dog, made in the prepubic location. The bilobed nature of the prostate, which is in cross section, can be seen.

1 Left lobe of prostate
2 Right lobe of prostate
3 Neck of urinary bladder

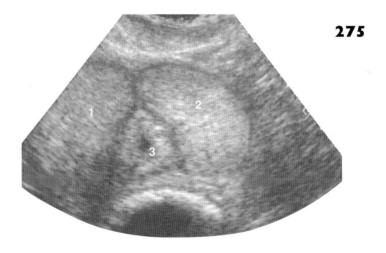

275

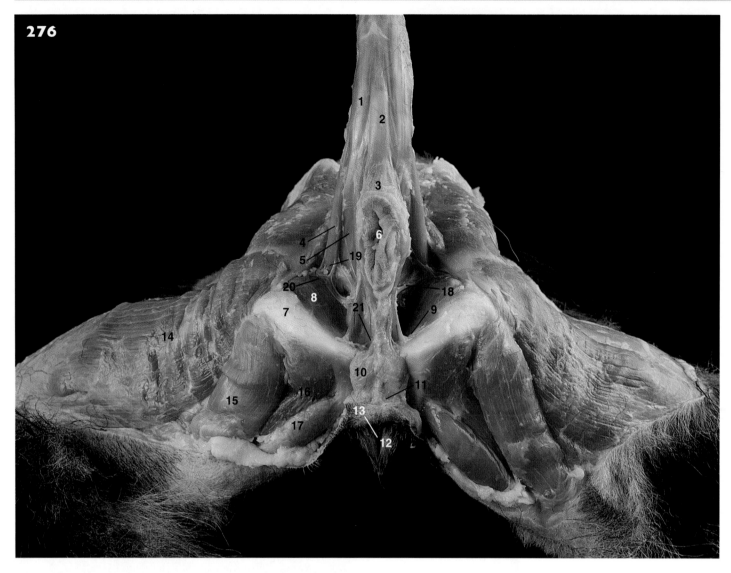

276

276   Caudal aspect of the perineum of a bitch.

1 M. sacrocaudalis ventralis lateralis	8 M. obturatorius internus	16 M. semimembranosus
2 M. rectococcygeus	9 M. ischiourethralis	17 M. gracilis
3 M. sphincter ani externus	10 M. constrictor vestibuli	18 Internal pudendal artery and vein, and pudendal nerve
4 M. coccygeus	11 M. constrictor vulvae	19 Caudal rectal artery and vein
5 M. levator ani	12 Labia	20 Perineal artery and vein
6 Anus	13 Vulva	21 Artery and vein of vestibular bulb
7 Ischiatic tuberosity	14 M. biceps femoris	
	15 M. semitendinosus	

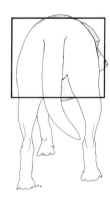

277   Caudolateral aspect of the perineum and external genitalia of a bitch.

1   M. gluteus medius
2   M. gluteus superficialis
3   Cranial dorsal iliac spine
4   M. sartorius
5   M. tensor fascia latae
6   Fascia lata
7   M. biceps femoris
8   M. semitendinosus
9   M. semimembranosus
10 Ischiatic tuberosity
11 Mm. intertransversarii
     dorsales caudales
12 Mm. intertransversarii
     ventrales caudales
13 Sacrotuberous ligament
14 M. coccygeus
15 M. levator ani
16 Anus
17 M. sphincter ani externus
18 Fibres from first and second
     caudal spinal nerves
19 M. constrictor vulvae
20 Vulva

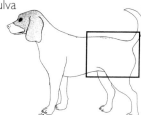

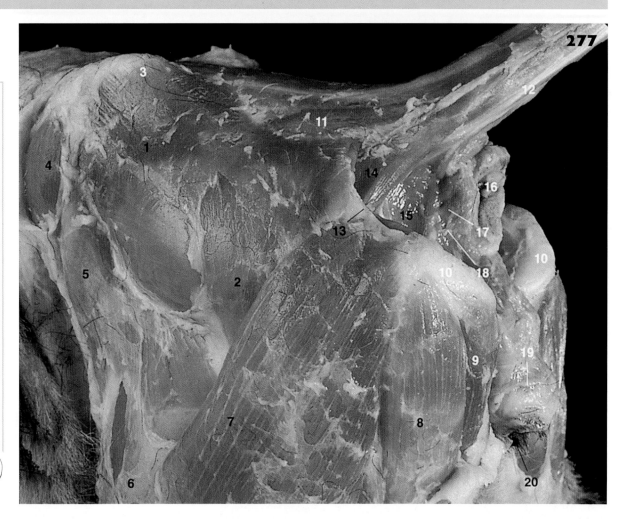

278   Caudal aspect of the perineum and external genitalia of a male dog.

1   M. rectococcygeus
2   M. sphincter ani externus
3   M. coccygeus
4   M. levator ani
5   Anus
6   Ischiatic tuberosity
7   M. obturatorius internus
8   Internal pudendal artery and
     vein, and pudendal nerve
9   M. ischiourethralis
10 M. ischiocavemosus
11 M. bulbospongiosus
12 M. retractor penis
13 M. biceps femoris
14 M. semitendinosus
15 M. semimembranosus
16 M. gracilis
17 M. adductor
18 Spermatic cord
19 Testis within parietal vaginal
     tunic
20 External spermatic fascia

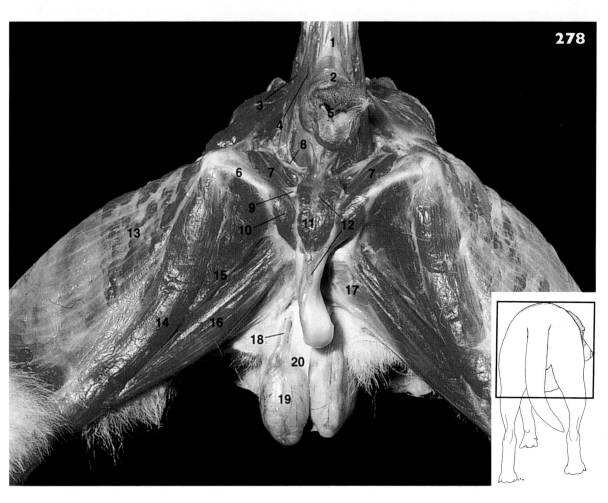

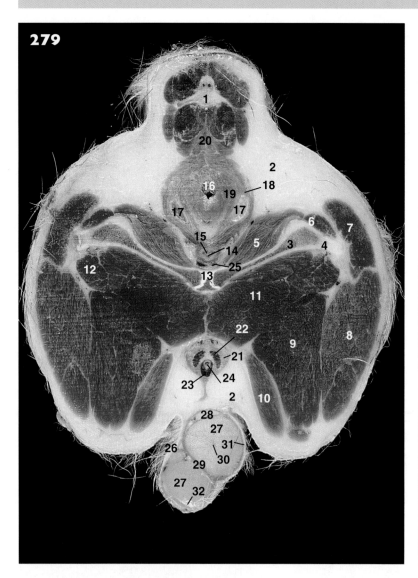

279

279   Caudal aspect of a transverse section through the perineal region of a dog at the level of the fourth caudal vertebra.

1	Fourth caudal vertebra	18	M. sphincter ani externus
2	Adipose tissue	19	M. sphincter ani internus
3	Ischium	20	M. rectococcygeus
4	Ischiatic tuberosity	21	Tunica albuginea of penis
5	M. gemellus	22	Corpus cavernosus penis
6	M. obturator internus	23	Corpus spongiosum
7	M. biceps femoris	24	Penile urethra
8	M. semitendinosus	25	Artery of penis
9	M. semimembranosus	26	Scrotum
10	M. gracilis	27	Testes
11	M. adductor	28	Epididymus
12	M. quadratus femoris	29	Scrotal septum
13	Pelvic symphysis	30	Mediastinum testis
14	Pelvic urethra	31	Vaginal tunic (parietal and
15	Pars spongiosum of urethra		visceral)
16	Anal canal	32	Spermatic fascia
17	Anal sacs		

Clinical Note

17   Note the position of the anal sacs lying between the internal and external sphincter muscles. The sac accumulates secretion from glands within its walls and this travels to the exterior via ducts opening at the periphery of the anal orifice. Blockage of these ducts can cause impaction of these sacs producing discomfort to the dog and even resulting in abcessation in the perineal region. Impaction can be relieved by digital pressure being applied laterally over the sacs resulting in expression of a foul-smelling secretion. The secretion is thought to be a scent-marking device of the dog.

280   Caudolateral aspect of the perineum of a male dog.

1   Cranial dorsal iliac spine
2   M. gluteus medius
3   M. gluteus superficialis
4   M. sartorius
5   M. tensor fasciae latae
6   Greater trochanter
7   M. biceps femoris
8   M. semitendinosus
9   M. semimembranosus
10 M. gracilis
11 Ischiatic tuberosity
12 Sacrotuberous ligament
13 Mm. intertransversarii dorsales caudales
14 Mm. intertransversarii ventrales caudales
15 M. coccygeus
16 M. levator ani
17 Anus
18 M. sphincter ani externus
19 Position of anal sac (deep to 18)
20 M. rectococcygeus
21 Fibres from first and second caudal spinal nerves
22 M. retractor penis
23 M. bulbospongiosus
24 M. ischiocavernosus
25 M. ischiourethralis
26 Body of penis
27 Corpus spongiosum penis
28 M. obturatorius internus
29 Internal pudendal artery giving origin to dorsal artery of penis and ventral perineal artery
30 Caudal rectal artery
31 Pudendal nerve

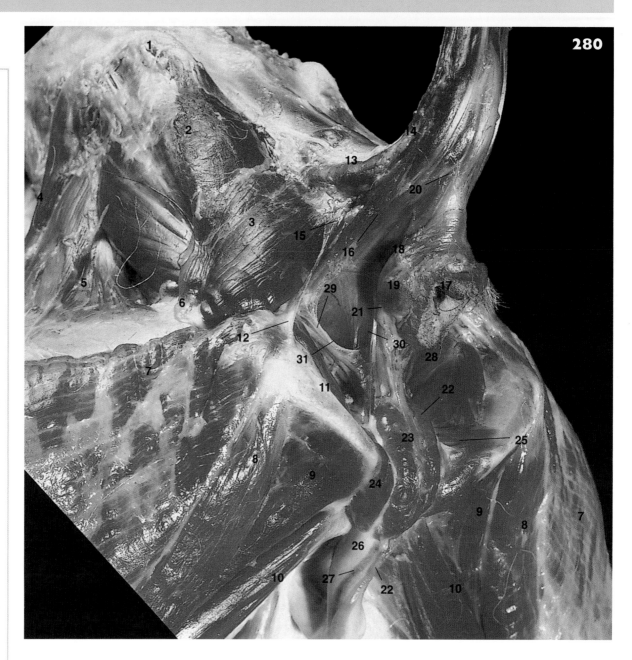

281   Dorsal (A) and ventral (B) aspect of the os penis of a dog.

1   Cranial extremity
2   Caudal extremity (proximal)
3   Ventral groove

Clinical Note
3   Note the ventral groove which encloses the urethra in life. Urethral obstruction commonly occurs at the proximal end of this groove.

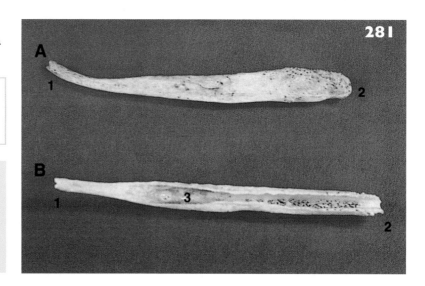

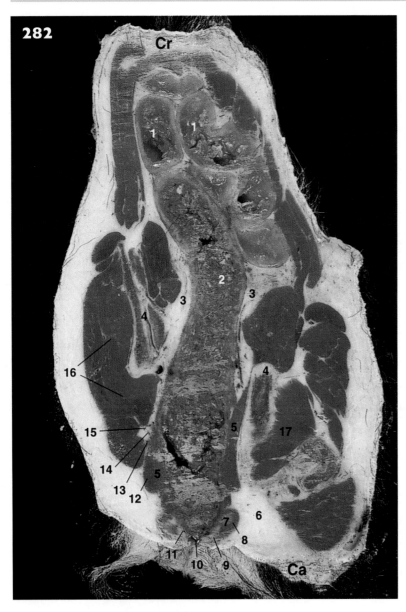

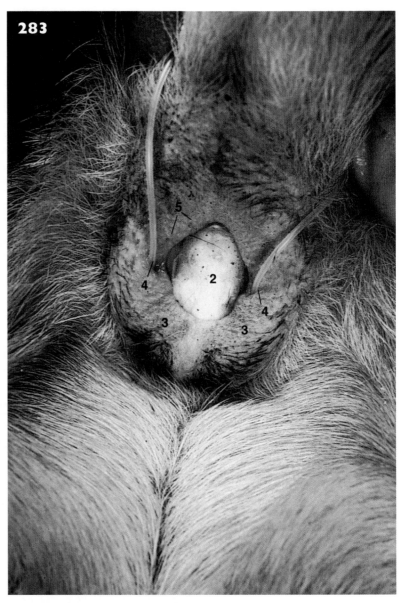

282   Dorsal aspect of a section made in the dorsal plane through the anus and pelvic cavity of a dog, showing the topography of the rectum and the muscles of the pelvic diaphragm. Orientation cranially (Cr) and caudally (Ca) is indicated.

1	Descending colon	10	Anal opening
2	Rectum	11	M. sphincter ani internus
3	Pelvic inlet	12	M. coccygeus
4	Ilium	13	Sacrotuberous ligament
5	M. levator ani	14	Ischiatic nerve
6	Fat (in ischiorectal fossa)	15	Caudal gluteal artery and vein
7	Anal sac	16	Gluteal muscle
8	M. sphincter ani externus	17	Mm. gemelli
9	Circumanal glands		

283   Caudal aspect of the anal region of a dog. The ducts of the anal sacs have been cannulated.

1	Tail	4	Opening of anal sac (cannulated)
2	Anus (with cotton plug)	5	Elevations for openings of
3	Cutaneous zone		circumanal glands

Clinical Note

13 & 14   Observe the relative proximity of the ischiatic nerve and the sacrotuberous ligament. In the repair of a perineal hernia, the ligament is used as an anchor point for suturing the muscles of the pelvic diaphragm, i.e. M. coccygeus (**12**) and M. levator ani (**5**), and entrapment of the ischiatic nerve is a potential hazard.

284   Radiograph of the abdominal region of a male dog in ventrodorsal positioning.

1 Costal arch
2 Thirteenth thoracic vertebra
3 Thirteenth (floating) rib
4 First lumbar vertebra
5 Seventh lumbar vertebra
6 Sacrum
7 Ilium
8 Femur
9 Os penis
10 Spinous process
11 Transverse process
12 Cranial articular process and mamillary process
13 Caudal articular process
14 Diaphragm
15 Stomach
16 Liver
17 Right kidney
18 Left kidney
19 Spleen
20 Jejunum
21 Caecum
22 Descending colon

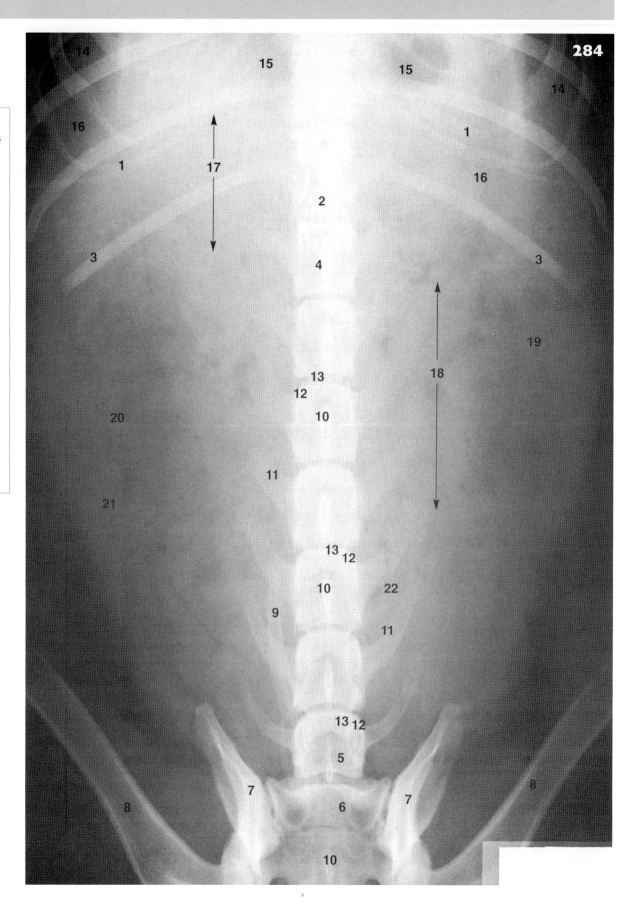

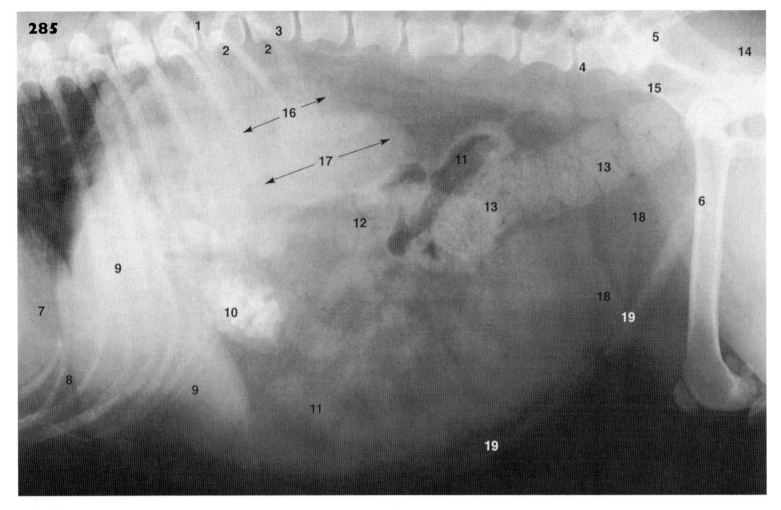

285   Radiograph of the abdominal region of a male dog in lateral recumbency.

1	Thirteenth thoracic vertebra	12	Region of ileocolic and
2	Thirteenth (floating) rib		caecolic junction
3	First lumbar vertebra	13	Descending colon
4	Seventh lumbar vertebra	14	Rectum
5	Sacrum	15	Wing of ilium
6	Femur	16	Right kidney (arrows)
7	Heart	17	Left kidney (arrows)
8	Diaphragm	18	Urinary bladder (distended,
9	Liver		intra-abdominal)
10	Stomach	19	Ventral abdominal wall
11	Jejunum		

286   Radiograph of the lateral aspect of the thorax and abdomen of a dog. Barium has been administered by mouth, and is seen in the upper digestive tract.

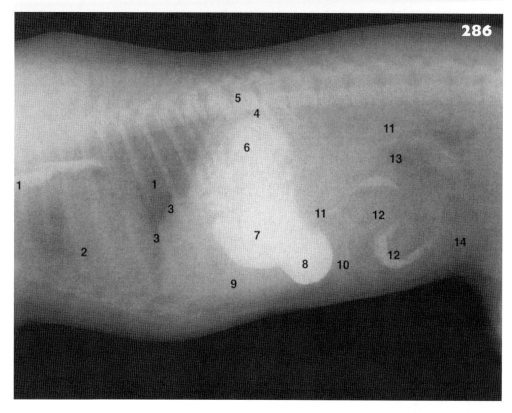

1 Oesophagus
2 Heart
3 Diaphragm
4 Thirteenth (floating) rib
5 Thirteenth thoracic vertebra
6 Fundus ⎫
7 Body ⎬ of stomach
8 Pyloric antrum ⎭
9 Liver
10 Spleen
11 Duodenum
12 Jejunum
13 Caecum
14 Abdominal wall

287   Ventrodorsal radiograph of the abdominal region of a dog in dorsal recumbency. Barium is lying intermingled with air in the stomach. The duodenum is outlined by barium filling, demonstrating the typical villous lining.

1 Diaphragm
2 Liver
3 Thirteenth (floating) rib
4 Cardia
5 Fundus (with barium) ⎫
6 Body (with air and barium) ⎬ of stomach
7 Pyloric antrum ⎭
8 Pylorus
9 Descending duodenum
10 Ascending duodenum
11 Jejunum
12 Ileum

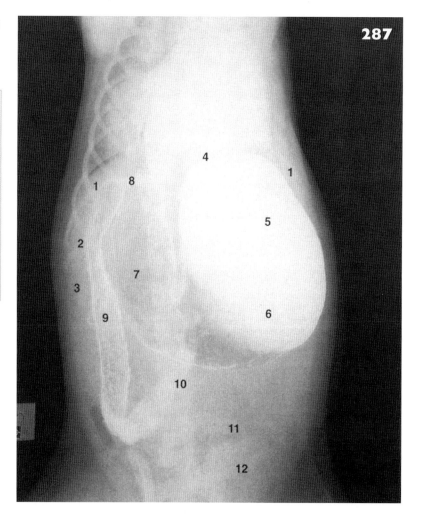

7 PELVIC LIMB

Working from the proximal pelvic region distally to the pes, the osteological details of each area of the pelvic limb are illustrated using bones, displayed both singly and in an articulated form, and radiographs. The relevant musculature is then exhibited. Contrast arteriograms and venograms are used to give an overview of the vascular supply, while nerve trunks are named where they appear in the dissected specimens.

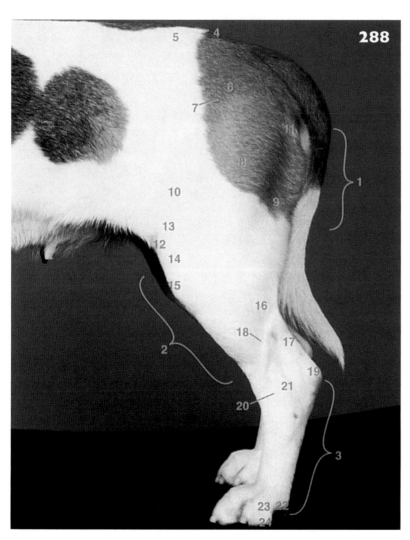

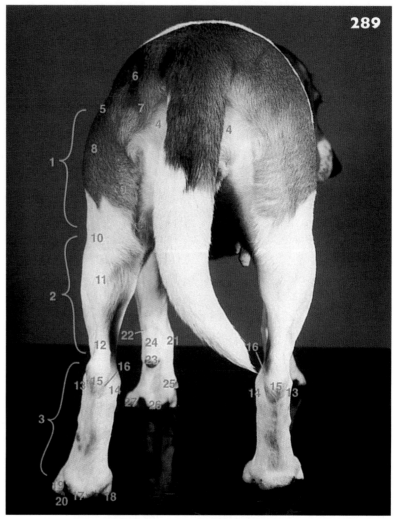

288 Lateral aspect of the left pelvic limb of a standing live dog, demonstrating palpable landmarks.

289 Caudal aspect of a standing live dog, demonstrating palpable landmarks. The palmar aspect of the manus of the thoracic limb is also shown.

1	Femoral region (thigh)	14	Stifle joint
2	Crus	15	Tibial tuberosity
3	Pes	16	M. gastrocnemius
4	Median crest of sacrum	17	Tendo calcaneus communis
5	Cranial dorsal iliac spine		(Achilles)
6	Greater trochanter	18	Lateral saphenous vein (site of
7	Level of hip joint		intravenous injection)
8	M. biceps femoris	19	Calcaneal tuberosity
9	M. semitendinosus	20	Tarsal joint (hock)
10	M. quadriceps femoris	21	Lateral malleolus of fibula
11	Ischiatic tuberosity	22	Metatarsal pad
12	Patella	23	Fifth digit
13	Lateral epicondyle of femur	24	Digital pad

Clinical Note

5, 6 & 11 These palpable bony prominences are used to verify the symmetry of the pelvic girdle during clinical examination for fracture of the ossa coxae or hip dislocation. The relative position of the three landmarks is compared on both sides.

1	Femoral region (thigh)	15	Calcaneal tuberosity	
2	Crus	16	Tarsal joint (hock)	
3	Pes	17	Metatarsal pad	
4	Perineum	18	Second digit	
5	Greater trochanter	19	Fifth digit	
6	Gluteal muscle mass	20	Digital pad	
7	Ischiatic tuberosity	21	Medial styloid	⎫
8	M. biceps femoris		process of radius	
9	M. semitendinosus	22	Carpal joint	
10	Stifle joint	23	Carpal pad	
11	M. gastrocnemius and	24	Accessory carpal	thoracic
	M. flexor digitorum superficialis		bone	limb
12	Tendo calcaneus communis	25	First digit (dew	
	(Achilles)		claw)	
13	Lateral malleolus of fibula	26	Metacarpal pad	
14	Medial malleolus of tibia	27	Fifth digit	⎭

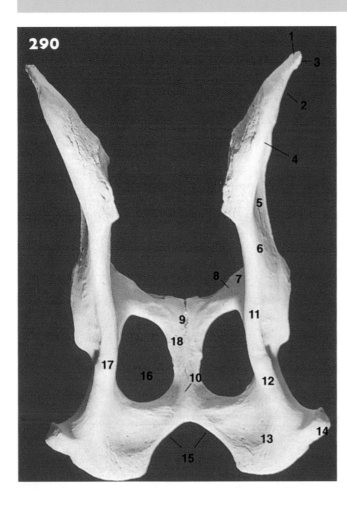

290   Dorsal aspect of the fused ossa coxae of a dog.

1 Iliac crest
2 Wing of ilium
3 Cranial dorsal iliac spine
4 Caudal dorsal iliac spine
5 Body of ilium
6 Greater ischiatic notch
7 Iliopubic eminence
8 Pecten of pubic bone
9 Symphysis pubis
10 Symphysis ischii
11 Ischiatic spine
12 Lesser ischiatic notch
13 Ischiatic table
14 Ischiatic tuberosity
15 Ischiatic arch
16 Obturator foramen
17 Grooves for M. obturatorius internus
18 Pubis

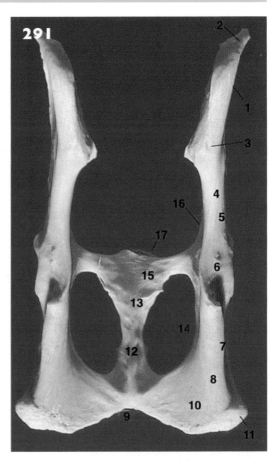

291   Dorsal aspect of the fused ossa coxae of a cat.

1 Wing of Ilium		10 Ischiatic table	
2 Cranial dorsal iliac spine		11 Ischiatic tuberosity	
3 Caudal dorsal iliac spine		12 Symphysis ischii	symphysis
4 Body of ilium		13 Symphysis pubis	pelvis
5 Greater ischiatic notch		14 Obturator foramen	
6 Ischiatic spine		15 Pubis	
7 Lesser ischiatic notch		16 Arcuate line	
8 Ischium		17 Pecten of pubic bone	
9 Ischiatic arch			

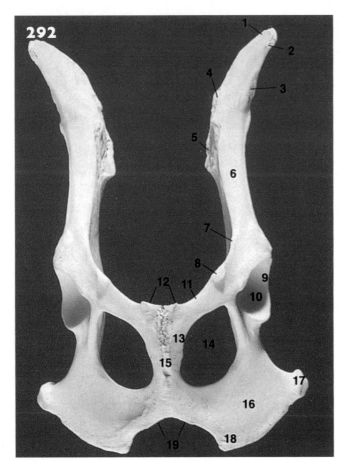

292   Ventral aspect of the fused ossa coxae of a dog.

1 Iliac crest	11 Pecten of pubic bone
2 Cranial ventral iliac spine	12 Pubic tubercle
3 Caudal ventral iliac spine	13 Pubis
4 Iliac tuberosity	14 Obturator foramen
5 Auricular surface	15 Symphysis pelvis
6 Body of Ilium	16 Ischium
7 Arcuate line	17 Ischiatic tuberosity
8 Iliopubic eminence	18 Medial angle of 17
9 Lunate surface of acetabulum	19 Ischiatic arch
10 Acetabular fossa	

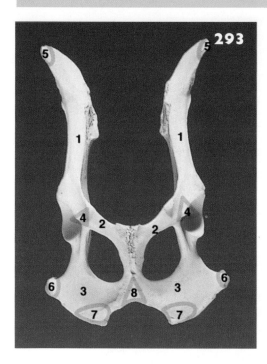

293   Ventral aspect of the fused ossa coxae of a dog, showing the centres of ossification.

1 Body of ilium	5 Iliac crest
2 Body of pubis	6 Ischiatic tuberosity
3 Body of ischium	7 Ischiatic arch
4 Acetabular bone	8 Symphysis

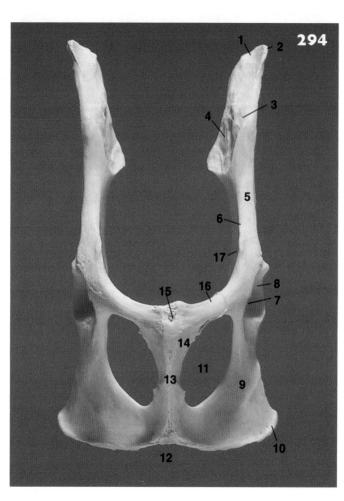

294   Ventral aspect of the fused ossa coxae of a cat.

1 Iliac crest	10 Ischiatic tuberosity
2 Cranial ventral iliac spine	11 Obturator foramen
3 Caudal ventral iliac spine	12 Ischiatic arch
4 Auricular surface	13 Symphysis pelvis
5 Body of ilium	14 Pubis
6 Arcuate line	15 Pubic tubercle
7 Acetabular fossa	16 Pecten of pubic bone
8 Lunate surface of acetabulum	17 Iliopubic eminence
9 Body of ischium	

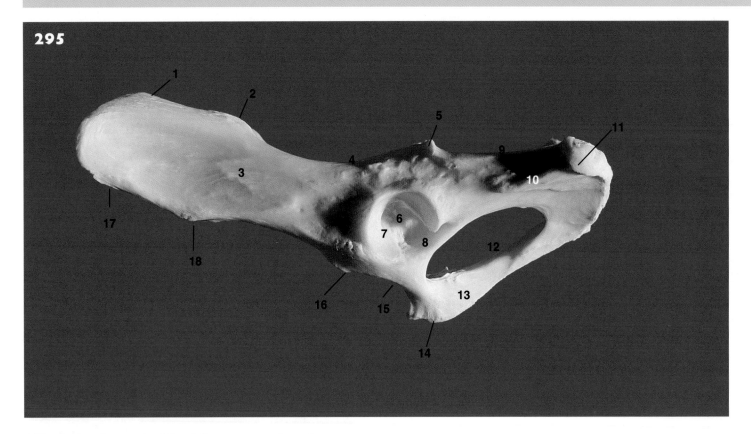

295   Lateral aspect of the left os coxae of a cat.

1	Cranial dorsal iliac spine	10	Body of ischium
2	Caudal dorsal iliac spine	11	Ischiatic tuberosity
3	Body of ilium	12	Obturator foramen
4	Greater ischiatic notch	13	Pubis
5	Ischiatic spine	14	Pubic tubercle
6	Acetabular fossa	15	Pecten of pubic bone
7	Lunate surface of acetabulum	16	Iliopubic eminence
8	Acetabular incisura	17	Cranial ventral iliac spine
9	Lesser ischiatic notch	18	Caudal ventral iliac spine

296   Lateral aspect of the left os coxae (A) and medial aspect of the right os coxae (B) of a dog.

1	Iliac crest
2	Cranial dorsal iliac spine
3	Caudal dorsal iliac spine
4	Wing
5	Gluteal surface } of ilium
6	Body
7	Greater ischiatic notch
8	Ischiatic spine
9	Ischium
10	Ischiatic tuberosity
11	Lesser ischiatic notch
12	Obturator foramen
13	Acetabular fossa
14	Lunate surface of acetabulum
15	Pubis
16	Pubic tubercle
17	Pecten of pubic bone
18	Iliopubic eminence
19	Tuberosity for M. rectus femoris
20	Caudal ventral iliac spine
21	Cranial ventral iliac spine
22	Iliac tuberosity
23	Sacroiliac joint
24	Iliac tuberosity
25	Auricular surface
26	Cranial dorsal iliac spine
27	Caudal dorsal iliac spine
28	Body of ilium
29	Greater ischiatic notch
30	Ischiatic spine
31	Grooves for M. obturatorius internus
32	Ischiatic tuberosity
33	Ischiatic table
34	Symphysis pelvis
35	Obturator foramen
36	Pubic tubercle
37	Pectin of pubic bone
38	Iliopubic eminence
39	Arcuate line
40	Caudal ventral iliac spine
41	Cranial ventral iliac spine

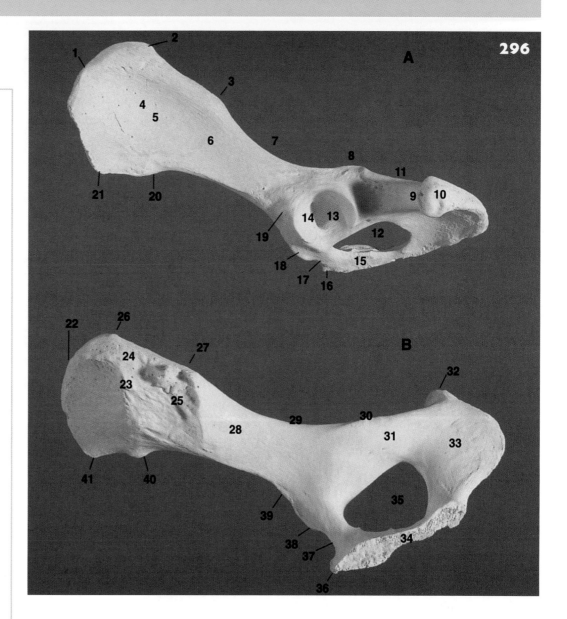

297   Lateral aspect of the left os coxae (A) and medial aspect of the right os coxae (B) of a dog, showing areas of muscle attachment.

1	Middle gluteal	13	Obturatorius externus
2	Sartorius	14	Adductor and gracilis
3	Tensor fasciae latae	15	Rectus abdominis
4	Deep gluteal	16	Pectineus
5	Iliacus	17	Psoas minor
6	Rectus femoris	18	Iliocostalis and longissimus lumborum
7	Articularis coxae	19	Quadratus lumborum
8	Gemelli	20	Coccygeus
9	Biceps femoris	21	Levator ani
10	Semitendinosus	22	Obturatorius internus
11	Semimembranosus	23	Ischiocavernosus
12	Quadratus femoris		

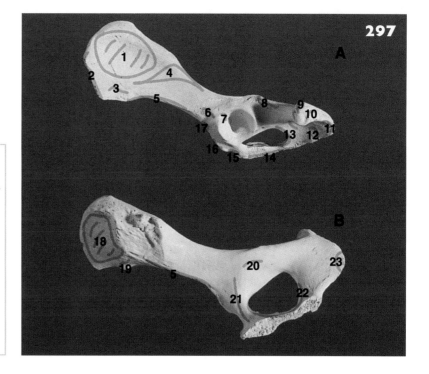

298

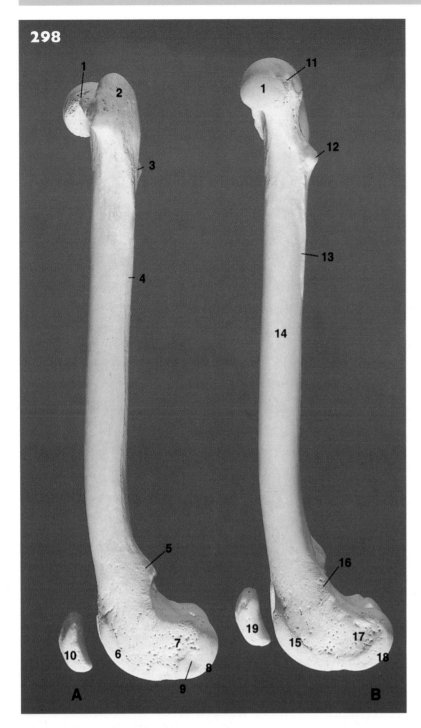

298   Lateral aspect of the left femur (A) and medial aspect of the right femur (B) of a dog.

1	Head	10	Patella
2	Greater trochanter	11	Fovea
3	Third trochanter (rudimentary)	12	Lesser trochanter
4	Lateral lip	13	Medial lip
5	Lateral supracondylar tuberosity	14	Body
6	Lateral trochlear ridge	15	Medial trochlear ridge
7	Lateral epicondyle	16	Medial supracondylar tuberosity
8	Lateral condyle	17	Medial epicondyle
9	Extensor fossa	18	Medial condyle
		19	Patella

299

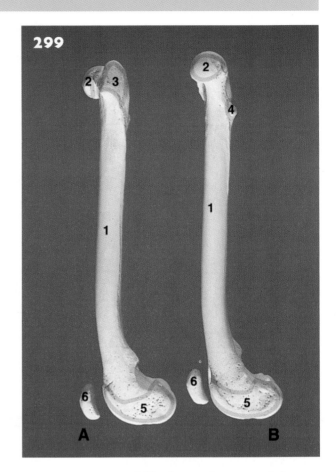

299   Lateral aspect of the left femur (A) and medial aspect of the right femur (B) of a dog, showing the centres of ossification.

1	Body of femur
2	Proximal
3	Greater trochanter
4	Lesser trochanter
5	Distal
6	Patella

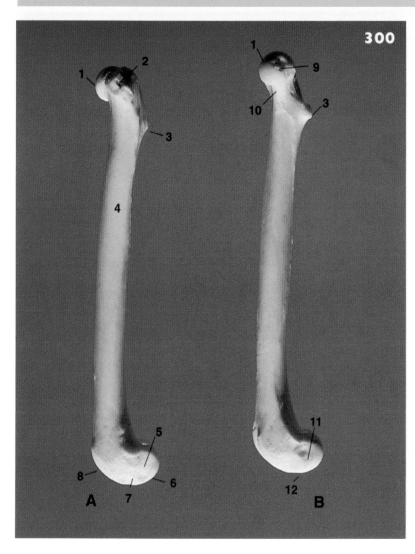

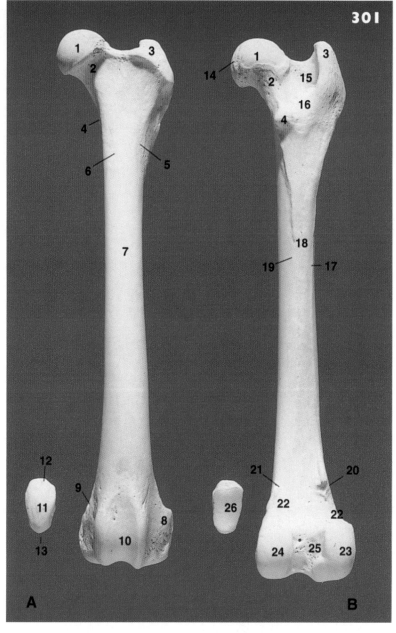

300 **Lateral aspect of the left femur (A) and medial aspect of the right femur (B) of a cat.**

1	Head	7	Extensor fossa
2	Greater trochanter	8	Trochlea
3	Lesser trochanter	9	Fovea
4	Body	10	Neck
5	Lateral epicondyle	11	Medial epicondyle
6	Lateral condyle	12	Medial condyle

301 **Cranial aspect of the left femur (A) and caudal aspect of the right femur (B) of a dog. The cranial and caudal aspects of the patella are also displayed.**

1	Head	15	Trochanteric fossa
2	Neck	16	Intertrochanteric crest
3	Greater trochanter	17	Lateral lip
4	Lesser trochanter	18	Roughened facie (facies aspera)
5	Line of M. vastus lateralis	19	Medial lip
6	Line of M. vastus medialis	20	Lateral supracondylar tuberosity
7	Body	21	Medial supracondylar tuberosity
8	Lateral epicondyle	22	Area of articulation of sesamoids (fabellae)
9	Medial epicondyle	23	Lateral condyle
10	Trochlea	24	Medial condyle
11	Patella	25	Intercondylar fossa
12	Base	26	Articular surface of patella
13	Apex		
14	Fovea		

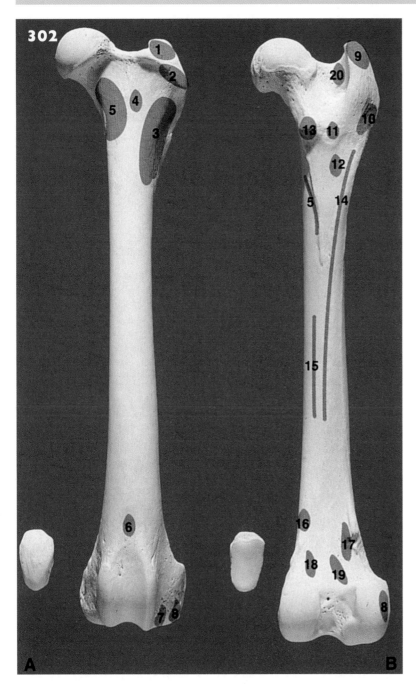

302   Cranial aspect of the left femur (A) and caudal aspect of the right femur (B) of a dog, showing areas of muscle attachment.

1	Gluteus medius	11	Quadratus femoris
2	Gluteus profundus	12	Adductor longus
3	Vastus lateralis and intermedius	13	Iliopsoas
4	Articularis coxae	14	Adductor magnus and brevis
5	Vastus medialis	15	Pectineus
6	Articularis genus	16	Semimembranosus
7	Flexor digitorum longus	17	Lateral head ⎱ of
8	Popliteus	18	Medial head ⎰ gastrocnemius
9	Piriformis and gluteus medius	19	Flexor digitorum superficialis
10	Gluteus superficialis	20	Gemelli and obturatorius internus and externus

303 Cranial aspect (A) of the left femur and caudal aspect (B) of the right femur of a cat.

1	Head	11	Fovea
2	Neck	12	Trochanteric fossa
3	Greater trochanter	13	Greater trochanter
4	Body	14	Lesser trochanter
5	Line of M. vastus lateralis	15	Intertrochanteric crest
6	Medial epicondyle	16	Popliteal surface
7	Lateral epicondyle	17	Medial condyle
8	Trochlea	18	Lateral condyle
9	Base ⎱ of patella	19	Intercondylar fossa
10	Apex ⎰	20	Articular surface of patella

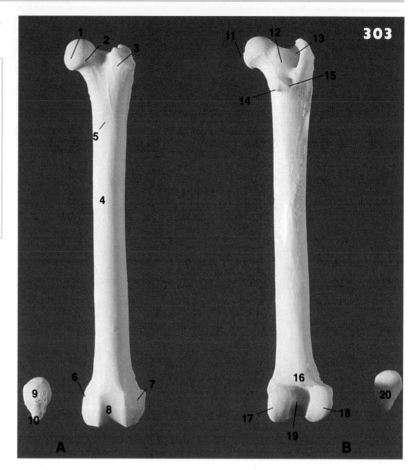

304 Proximal and distal extremities of the femur of a dog.

1	Fovea	6	Intertrochanteric crest
2	Head	7	Trochlea
3	Greater trochanter	8	Intercondylar fossa
4	Trochanteric fossa	9	Lateral condyle
5	Lesser trochanter	10	Medial condyle

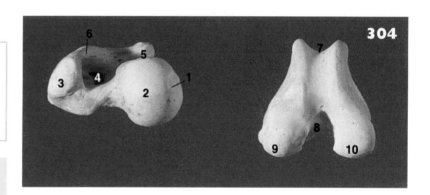

Clinical Note
4 This is the point at which an intramedullary pin is withdrawn and reinserted during reverse intramedullary pinning of a fractured femur. Because of the eccentric placement of the articular surface of the femoral head relative to the longitudinal dimension of the femoral body (Fig. 301, **1, 2 & 7**), it is possible to use a reverse pinning technique on the femur.

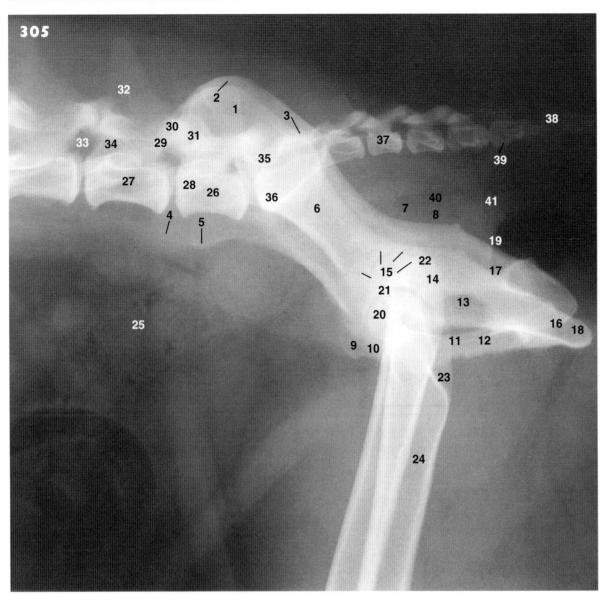

305

1   Wing of ilium
2   Cranial dorsal iliac spine
3   Caudal dorsal iliac spine
4   Cranial ventral iliac spine
5   Caudal ventral iliac spine
6   Body of ilium
7   Greater ischiatic notch
8   Ischiatic spine
9   Iliopectineal eminence
10 Pecten of pubis
11 Pubis
12 Symphysis pelvis
13 Obturator foramen
14 Acetabular notch
15 Acetabulum
16 Ischiatic arch
17 Ischiatic body
18 Ischiatic tuberosity
19 Lesser ischiatic notch
20 Head of femur
21 Hip joint
22 Greater trochanter
23 Lesser trochanter
24 Body of femur
25 Descending colon
26 Seventh lumbar vertebra
27 Body of sixth lumbar
    vertebra
28 Transverse process
29 Accessory process
30 Caudal articular process
31 Cranial articular process
32 Spinous process
33 Intervertebral foramen
34 Vertebral canal
35 Wing of sacrum
36 Promontory
37 First caudal vertebra
38 Fifth caudal vertebra
39 Haemal arch
40 Rectum
41 Anus

306   Ventrodorsal radiograph of the pelvis of a male dog.

1 Wing ⎱ of ilium
2 Body ⎰
3 Dorsal border
4 Ventral border
5 Caudal ventral iliac spine
6 Cranial ventral iliac spine
7 Iliac crest
8 Acetabular branch of pubis
9 Pecten of pubis
10 Iliopectineal eminence
11 Symphyseal branch of pubis
12 Symphyseal branch of ischium
13 Ischiatic table
14 Ischiatic tuberosity
15 Body of ischium
16 Lesser ischiatic notch
17 Ischiatic arch
18 Obturator foramen
19 Ischiatic spine
20 Dorsal acetabular border
21 Ventral acetabular border
22 Acetabular fossa and incisura
23 Cranial edge ⎱ of acetabular
24 Caudal edge ⎰ image
25 Head ⎱ of femur
26 Neck ⎰
27 Greater trochanter
28 Trochanteric fossa
29 Lesser trochanter
30 Body of femur
31 Descending colon
32 Body of seventh lumbar vertebra
33 Spinous process
34 Transverse process
35 Wing of sacrum
36 Rectum
37 Spinous process of sacrum
38 Outline of os penis

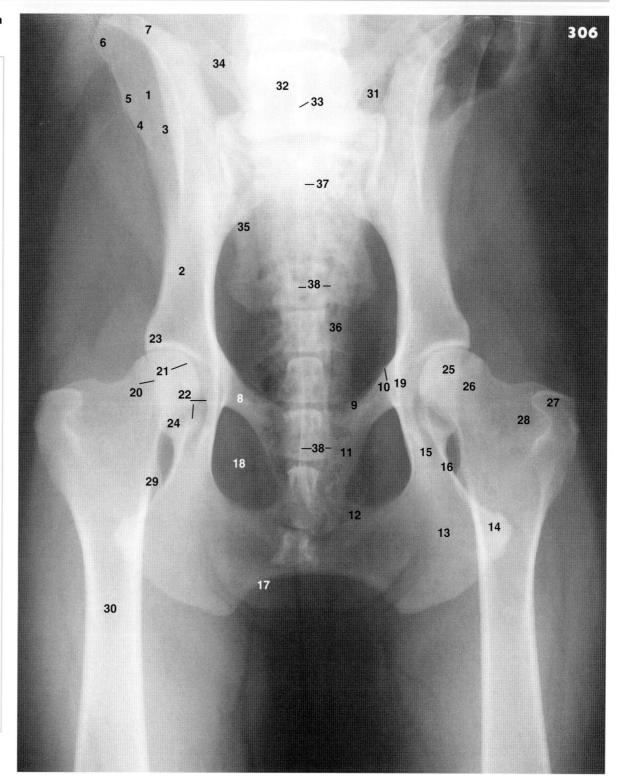

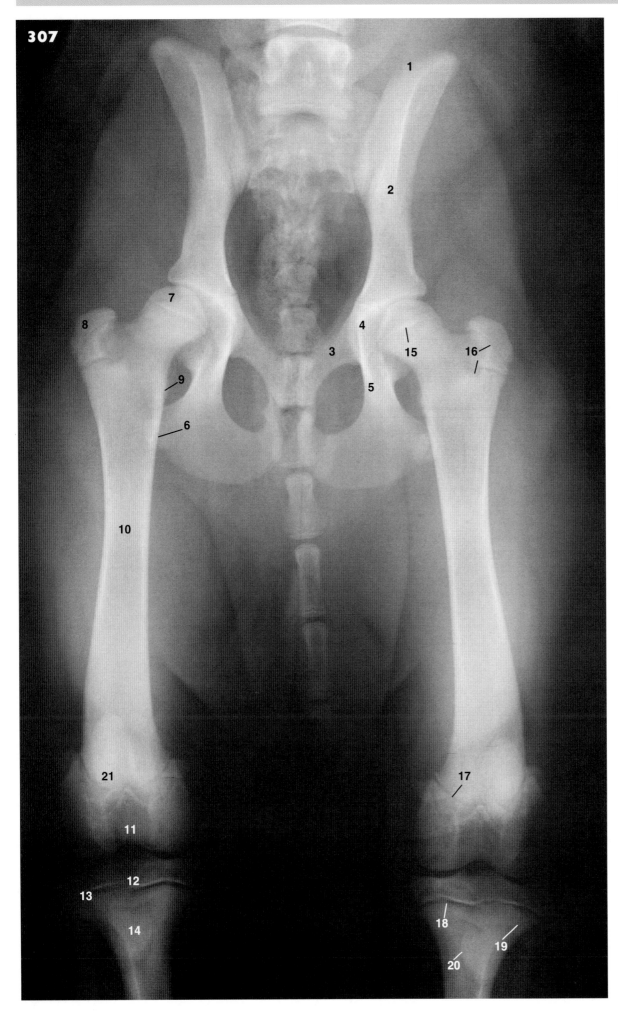

307

307 Ventrodorsal radiograph of the pelvis and stifles of a puppy, showing the centres of ossification.

1	Iliac crest
2	Body of ilium
3	Pubis
4	Acetabular bone
5	Body of ischium
6	Ischiatic tuberosity
7	Head of femur
8	Greater trochanter
9	Lesser trochanter
10	Body of femur
11	Distal femoral epiphysis
12	Proximal tibial epiphysis
13	Proximal fibular epiphysis
14	Tibial tuberosity
15	Proximal femoral growth plate
16	Growth plate for greater trochanter
17	Distal femoral growth plate
18	Proximal tibial growth plate
19	Proximal fibular growth plate
20	Growth plate for tibial tuberosity
21	Patella in trochlea

308 Ventrodorsal radiograph of the pelvis and pelvic limbs of a 19-week-old kitten showing the centres of ossification.

1 Cranial growth plate for the body of the seventh lumbar vertebra
2 Sacrum
3 Ilium
4 Ischium
5 Pubis
6 Body of second caudal vertebra
7 Obturator foramen
8 Acetabulum
9 Growth plate of acetabulum between bones 3, 4 and 5 and acetabular bone
10 Head of femur
11 Growth plate between the centre of ossification for the greater trochanter and the body of the femur
12 Lesser trochanter
13 Symphysis pelvis
14 Growth plate between the centre of ossification for the ischiatic tuberosity and the ischiatic table
15 Proximal femoral epiphysis
16 Body of femur
17 Distal femoral epiphysis
18 Patella
19 Fabella

20 Medial femoral condyle
21 Lateral femoral condyle
22 Proximal tibial epiphysis
23 Body of tibia
24 Growth plate between the body of tibia and the tibial tuberosity
25 Proximal fibular epiphysis
26 Body of fibula
27 Distal epiphysis of tibia
28 Distal epiphysis of fibula
29 Body of calcaneus
30 Centre of ossification for the calcaneal tuberosity
31 Talus
32 Distal row of tarsal bones
33 Second to fifth metatarsal bones
34 Distal epiphysis of metatarsal bone
35 Bony elements of first digit
36 Proximal sesamoid bones
37 Proximal epiphysis of proximal phalanx
38 Body of proximal phalanx
39 Proximal epiphysis of middle phalanx
40 Body of middle phalanx
41 Body of distal phalanx

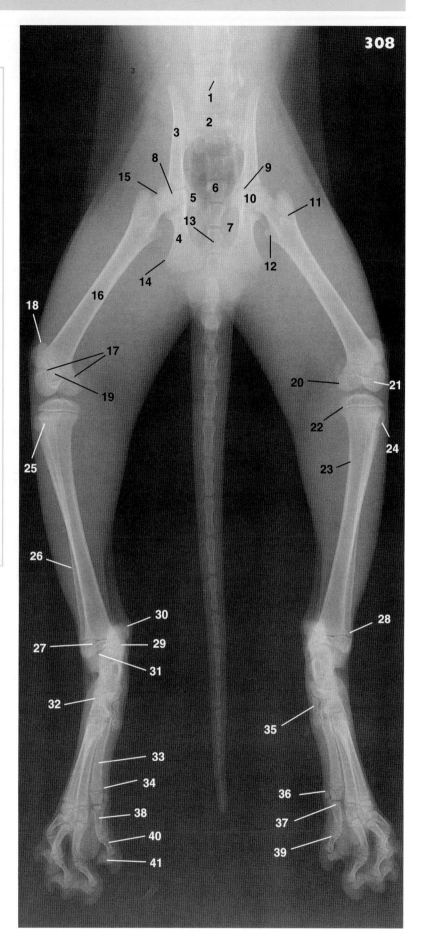

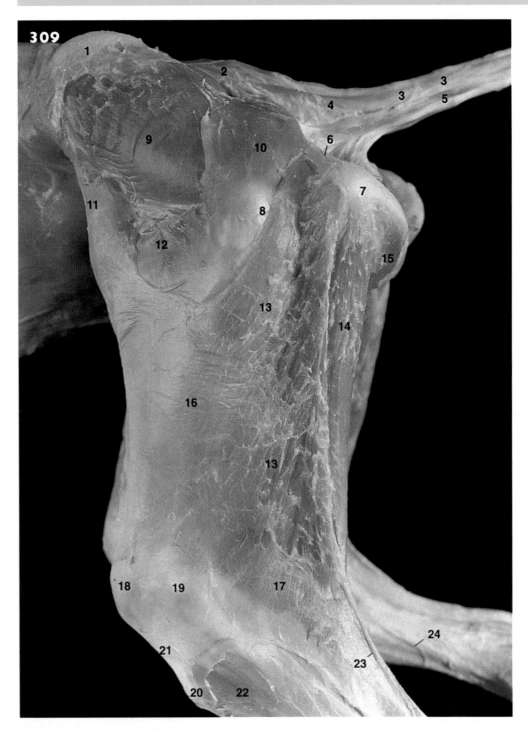

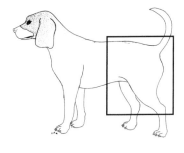

309 **Lateral aspect of the pelvic and thigh regions of the left pelvic limb of a dog. The skin has been removed to reveal the superficial muscles.**

1 Dorsal iliac spine	8 Greater trochanter	17 Continuation of M. biceps
2 Sacrum	9 M. gluteus medius	femoris
3 Caudal vertebrae	10 M. gluteus superficialis	18 Patella in trochlear groove
4 Mm. intertransversarii dorsales	11 M. sartorius	19 Lateral epicondyle of femur
caudalis	12 M. tensor fasciae latae	20 Tibial tuberosity
5 Mm. intertransversarii	13 M. biceps femoris	21 Patellar ligament
ventrales caudalis	14 M. semitendinosus	22 M. tibialis cranialis
6 Sacrotuberous ligament	15 M. semimembranosus	23 Lateral saphenous vein
7 Ischiatic tuberosity	16 Fascia lata extending to stifle	24 Medial saphenous vein

Clinical Note
16 This is the approach for exposing the midshaft of the femur. The incision is made along the line of fusion of the fascia lata and the cranial edge of the biceps femoris muscle.

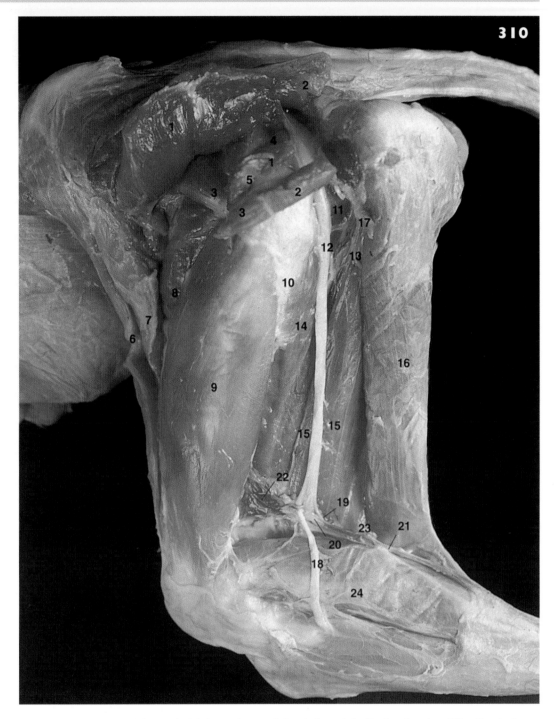

310

310   Lateral aspect of the pelvic and thigh regions of the left pelvic limb of a dog. The fascia lata and biceps femoris muscle have been removed to reveal the deeper muscles. The gluteal muscles have been reflected dorsally.

1 M. gluteus medius ⎫	
2 M. gluteus superficialis ⎬ (cut)	
3 M. gluteus profundus ⎭	
4 M. piriformis	
5 Hip joint capsule	
6 M. sartorius	
7 M. tensor fasciae latae	
8 M. rectus femoris	
9 M. vastus lateralis	

10 Femur	
11 M. quadratus femoris	
12 Ischiatic nerve	
13 Caudal gluteal artery and vein	
14 M. adductor	
15 M. semimembranosus	
16 M. semitendinosus	
17 M. abductor cruris caudalis	
(cut proximal end)	

18 Common peroneal (fibular) nerve	
19 Caudal cutaneous sural nerve	
20 Tibial nerve	
21 Lateral saphenous vein	
22 Femoral artery and vein	
23 Popliteal lymph node	
24 M. gastrocnemius	

Clinical Note

1, 2 & 3 The tendons of insertion of the gluteal muscles onto or over the greater trochanter have been sectioned in the manner used in a dorsal surgical approach to the hip joint.

12 Note the course of this nerve as it runs through the region caudal to the hip joint. The nerve must be identified and conserved during surgery of the hip joint.

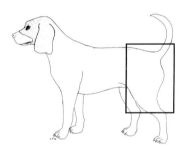

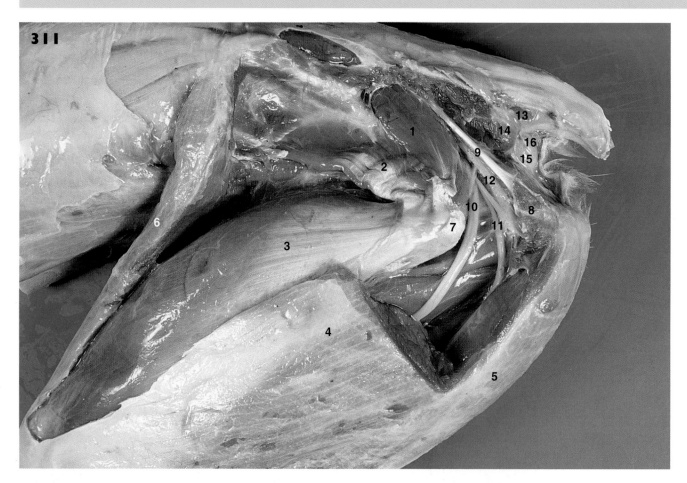

311

311   Lateral aspect of the pelvic region of the left pelvic limb of a dog. The superficial and middle gluteal muscles have been removed to reveal the deep gluteal muscle. The fascia lata and its tensor muscle along with the proximal segment of the biceps femoris muscle have been removed to reveal the quadriceps group of muscles.

1	M. piriformis	9	Sacrotuberous ligament
2	M. gluteus profundus	10	Ischiatic nerve
3	M. vastus lateralis	11	Branch of 10 running to 4 & 5
4	M. biceps femoris (cut)	12	Caudal gluteal artery and vein
5	M. semitendinosus	13	M. levator ani
6	M. sartorius	14	M. coccygeus
7	Greater trochanter	15	Position of anal sac
8	Ischiatic tuberosity	16	M. sphincter ani externus

Clinical Note

13 & 14   Note that these muscles lie lateral to the rectum as it becomes confluent with the anal canal. In this position they provide lateral support to the rectum during straining movements involved in the function of defaecation, forming the pelvic diaphragm. Breakdown of this muscular support can allow the rectum to deviate laterally to develop a perineal hernia. Surgical repair may be attempted to rebuild the lateral support. This involves sutures tying the muscles **13 & 14** to the sacrotuberous ligament (**9**). This procedure must be approached with caution due to the close approximation of the ligament to the ischiatic nerve trunk (**10**). If the sutures incorporate the nerve then paralysis of the ischiatic nerve may ensue with loss of motor function to the majority of the muscles of the pelvic limb.

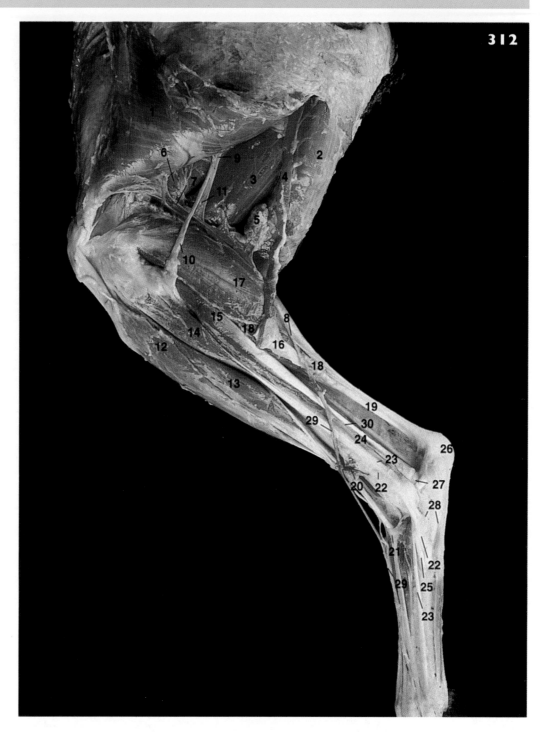

312

312 Lateral aspect of the left thigh, crus and tarsal region of a dog. The biceps femoris muscle has been reflected to reveal the division of the ischiatic nerve.

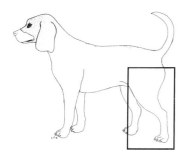

Clinical Note
5 This node is palpable in the normal dog during clinical examination. Enlargement of this node could indicate infection within the pelvic limb of that side.
29 & 30 The lateral saphenous vein is used for venepuncture in the dog as it lies on the lateral crural region. The medial saphenous nerve can also be used – this is more often used in the cat.

1	M. biceps femoris (reflected)	11	Tibial nerve
2	M. semitendinosus	12	M. tibialis cranialis
3	M. semimembranosus	13	M. extensor digitorum longus
4	M. abductor cruris caudalis	14	M. peroneus longus
5	Popliteal lymph node	15	M. flexor hallucis longus
6	Femoral artery and vein		(lateral head of M. flexor
7	Caudal femoral artery and		digitorum profundus)
	vein	16	Tendons of 1 and 2
8	Lateral saphenous vein	17	M. gastrocnemius
9	Ischiatic nerve	18	M. flexor digitorum superficialis
10	Common peroneal (fibular)	19	Tendo calcaneus communis
	nerve		(Achilles)

20	Proximal extensor retinaculum
21	Distal extensor retinaculum
22	Tendon of 14
23	Tendon of M. extensor
	digitorum lateralis
24	M. peroneus brevis
25	Tendon of 24
26	Calcaneal tuberosity
27	Short part | of lateral collateral
28	Long part | ligament of tarsus
29	Cranial ramus | of lateral
30	Caudal ramus | saphenous vein

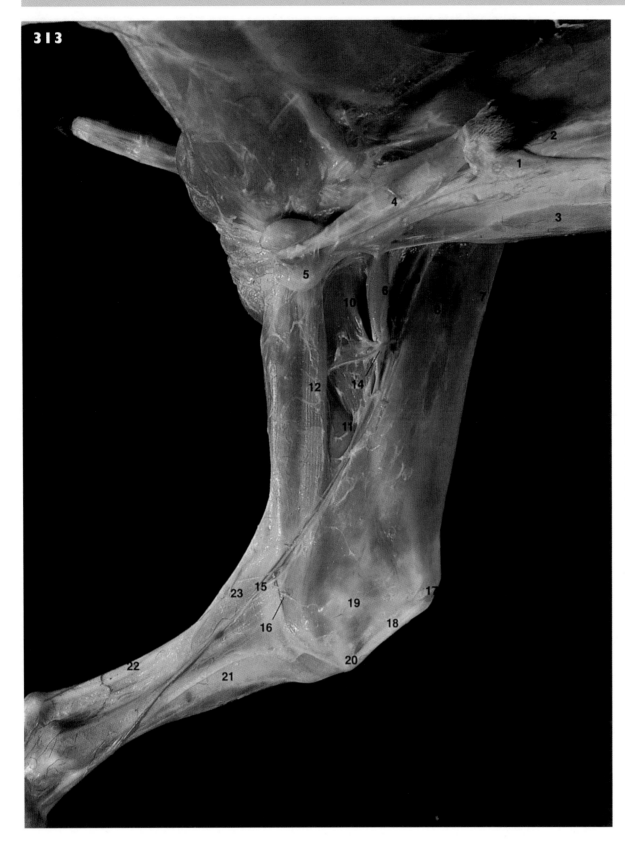

313 Medial aspect of the thigh region of the left pelvic limb of a dog, showing the superficial muscles.

1 M. preputialis
2 M. rectus abdominis
3 M. obliquus externus abdominis
4 Glans penis
5 Testes
6 M. pectineus
7 Cranial part } of M. sartorius
8 Caudal part }
9 M. rectus femoris
10 Mm. adductores
11 M. semimembranosus
12 M. gracilis
13 Femoral triangle (with femoral artery, vein and saphenous nerve)
14 Muscular branches
15 Medial saphenous vein
16 Middle genicular vein
17 Patella
18 Patellar ligament
19 Medial epicondyle of femur
20 Tibial tuberosity
21 Body of tibia
22 Tendo calcaneus communis (Achilles)
23 M. gastrocnemius

Clinical Note
13 It is in this position that the clinician places his fingers when taking the animal's pulse rate from the femoral artery. This is also a site for venepuncture in the anaesthetised dog when larger volumes of blood are required.

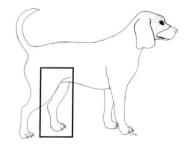

314 **Medial aspect of the thigh region and crus of the left pelvic limb of a dog. The limb has been resected from its body attachments, and the caudal part of the sartorius muscle has been cut to reveal the deeper muscles.**

1 M. sartorius
2 M. vastus medialis
3 M. adductor
4 M. semimembranosus
5 M. gracilis
6 M. semitendinosus
7 M. gastrocnemius
8 Saphenous artery, vein and nerve
9 M. popliteus
10 Medial collateral ligament of stifle
11 Patella
12 Patellar ligament
13 Tibial tuberosity
14 M. sartorius (cut end)
15 M. tibialis cranialis
16 M. flexor digitorum longus
17 M. flexor hallucis longus (lateral head of M. flexor digitorum profundus)
18 M. flexor digitorum superficialis
19 Tendons of 6 and M. biceps femoris (cut end)
20 Tendo calcaneus communis (Achilles)
21 Saphenous artery (caudal branch)
22 Tendon of 17
23 Tendon of 16
24 Body of tibia
25 Proximal extensor retinaculum
26 Tendon of 15
27 Medial collateral ligament of tarsus
28 Second metatarsal bone
29 Mm. interossei
30 Tendon of 18
31 Tendon of M. flexor digitorum profundus

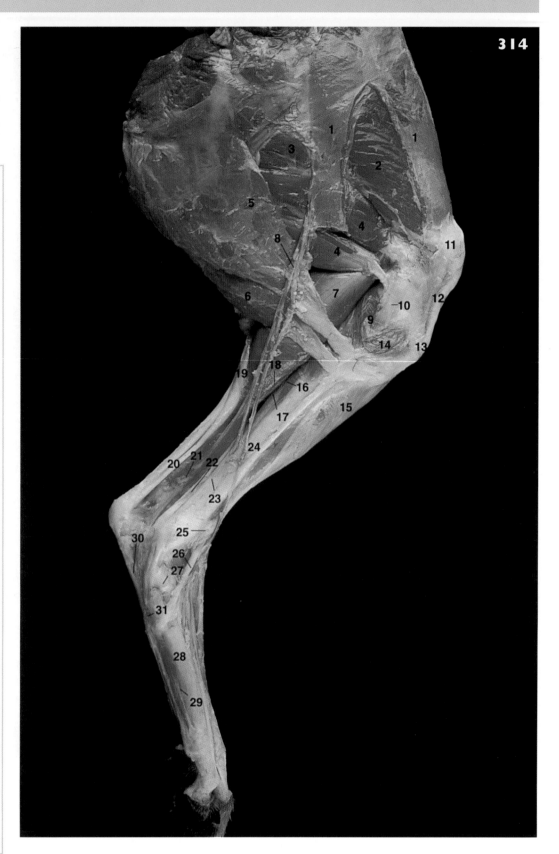

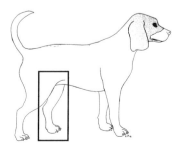

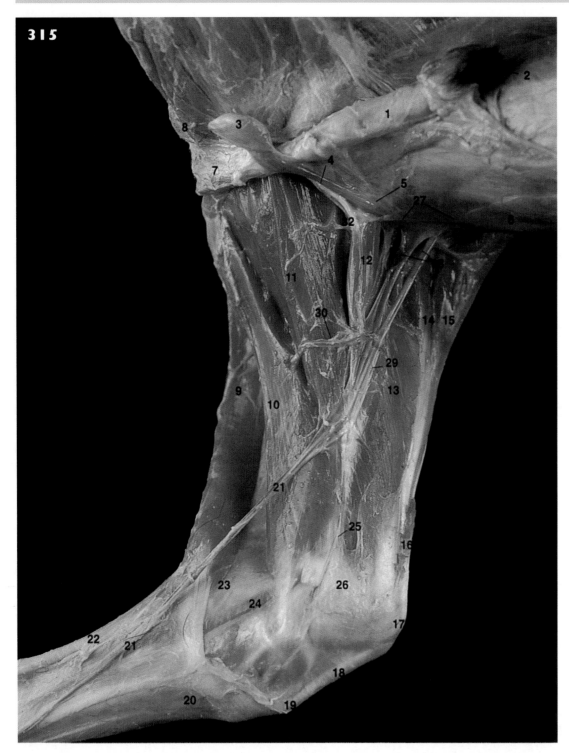

315

315   Medial aspect of the thigh region of the left pelvic limb of a dog. The gracilis and sartorius muscles have been resected.

1   Glans penis
2   External preputial orifice
3   Testis within parietal layer of vaginal tunic
4   Spermatic cord
5   Superficial (external) inguinal ring
6   M. obliquus externus abdominis
7   Body of penis
8   Ischiatic tuberosity
9   M. semitendinosus
10   M. semimembranosus
11   Mm. adductor magnus and brevis
12   M. pectineus
13   M. vastus medialis
14   M. rectus femoris
15   M. tensor fasciae latae
16   Fascia lata
17   Patella
18   Patellar ligament
19   Tibial tuberosity
20   Body of tibia
21   Medial saphenous artery and vein
22   Tendo calcaneus communis (Achilles)
23   M. gastrocnemius
24   M. popliteus
25   Middle genicular vein
26   Medial epicondyle of femur
27   Femoral triangle
28   Femoral artery and vein
29   Saphenous nerve (from femoral nerve)
30   Middle caudal femoral artery and vein
31   Branch of femoral nerve to 15 and M. sartorius
32   Branch of obturator nerve to M. pectineus and M. adductor

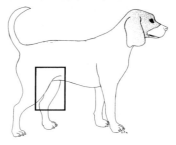

316   Medial aspect of the left crus of a dog.

1   M. semitendinosus
2   M. gastrocnemius
3   M. popliteus
4   Tendons of M. biceps femoris and 1 (cut end)
5   Saphenous artery and vein
6   M. flexor hallucis longus
7   M. flexor digitorum longus (medial head of M. flexor digitorum profundus)
8   Tendon of M. flexor hallucis longus (lateral head of M. flexor digitorum profundus)
9   M. tibialis cranialis
10   Body of tibia
11   Proximal extensor retinaculum
12   Tendo calcaneus communis (Achilles)
13   Calcaneal tuberosity
14   Tendon of M. tibialis caudalis
15   Medial collateral ligament
16   Tendon of M. flexor digitorum superficialis
17   Tendon of M. flexor digitorum profundus
18   Mm. interossei

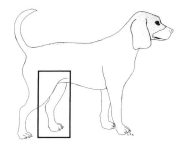

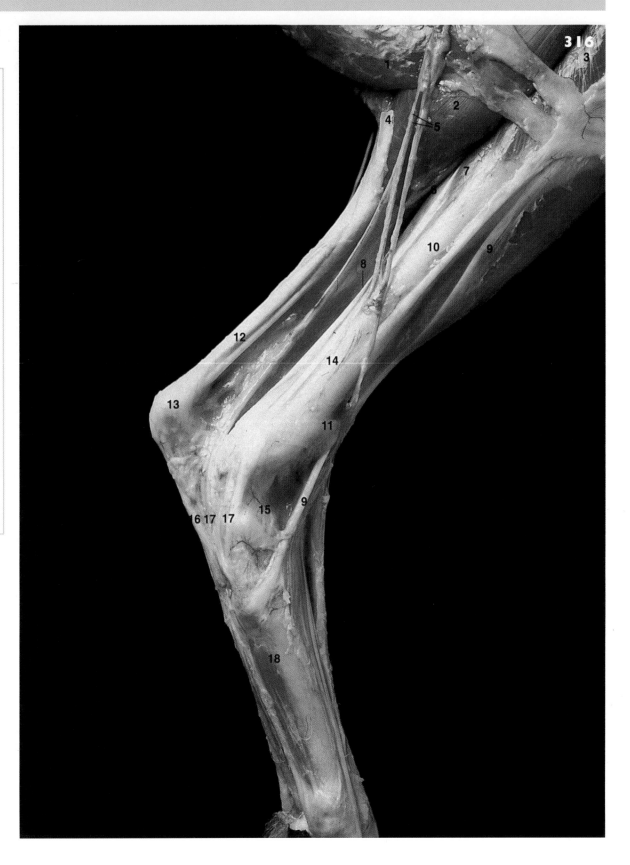

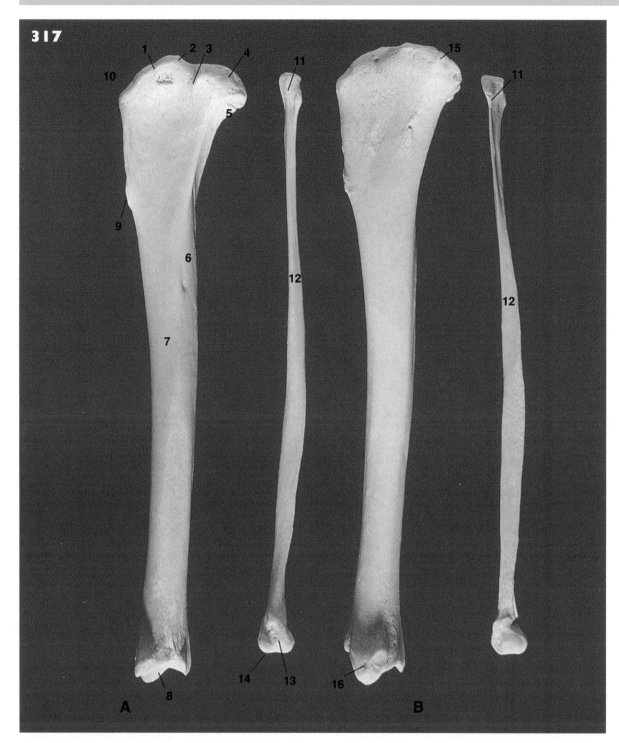

317   **Lateral aspect of the left tibia and fibula (A) and medial aspect of the right tibia and fibula (B) of a dog.**

1   Cranial intercondylar area
2   Intercondylar eminence
3   Muscular (extensor) groove
4   Lateral condyle
5   Facet for articulation with fibula
6   Interosseous border
7   Body of tibia
8   Distal articular surface with cochlea of tibia
9   Cranial border (tibial crest)
10 Tibial tuberosity
11 Head ⎱ of fibula
12 Body ⎰
13 Lateral malleolus
14 Groove of 13
15 Medial condyle
16 Medial malleolus

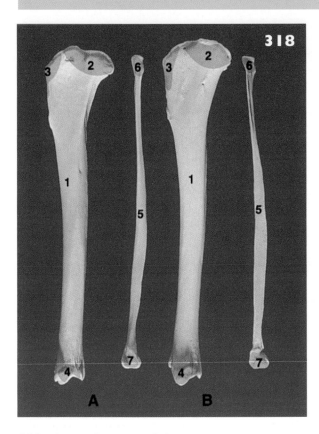

318 Lateral aspect of the left tibia and fibula (A) and medial aspect of the right tibia and fibula (B) of a dog, showing the centres of ossification.

1	Body of tibia
2	Proximal tibia
3	Tibial tuberosity
4	Distal tibia
5	Body of fibula
6	Proximal fibula
7	Distal fibula

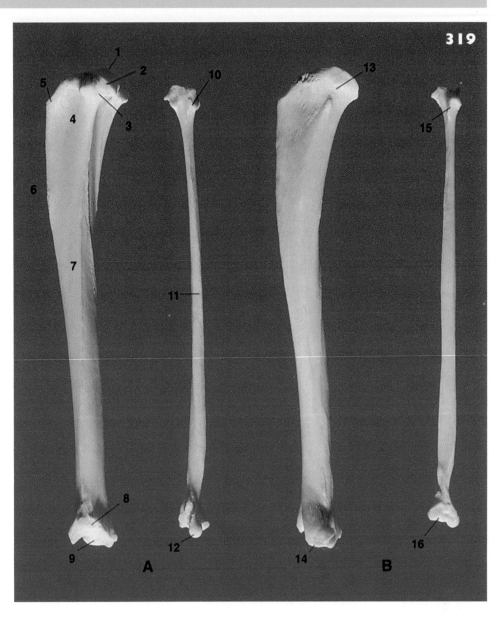

319 Lateral aspect of the left tibia and fibula (A) and medial aspect of the right tibia and fibula (B) of a cat.

1	Intercondylar eminence	9	Distal articular surface
2	Lateral condyle of tibia	10	Head ⎫ of fibula
3	Facet for proximal articulation with fibula	11	Body ⎭
4	Muscular groove	12	Lateral malleolus
5	Tibial tuberosity	13	Medial condyle of tibia
6	Cranial border (tibial crest)	14	Medial malleolus
7	Body of tibia	15	Facet for proximal articulation with tibia
8	Facet for distal articulation with fibula	16	Facet for distal articulation with tibia

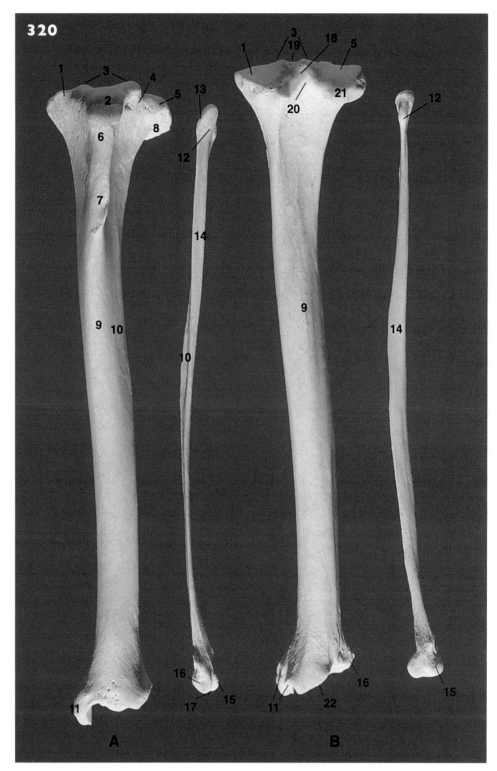

320 Cranial aspect of the left tibia and fibula **(A)** and caudal aspect of the right tibia and fibula **(B)** of a dog.

321 Cranial aspect of the left tibia and fibula **(A)** and caudal aspect of the right tibia and fibula **(B)** of a dog, showing areas of muscle attachment.

1	Biceps femoris
2	Cranial tibial
3	Peroneus longus
4	Quadriceps femoris
5	Sartorius
6	Gracilis
7	Semitendinosus
8	Flexor hallucis longus (radial)
9	Extensor digitorum lateralis
10	Extensor hallucis longus (ulnar)
11	Peroneus brevis
12	Caudal tibial (ulnar)
13	Flexor hallucis longus (lateral head of M. flexor digitorum profundus)
14	Caudal tibial (tibial)
15	Flexor digitorum longus (medial head of M. flexor digitorum profundus)
16	Popliteus

1	Medial condyle	9	Body of tibia	17	Groove of lateral malleolus (sulcus malleolaris lateralis)
2	Cranial intercondylar area	10	Interosseous border	18	Intercondylar eminence
3	Medial and lateral intercondylar tubercles	11	Medial malleolus	19	Caudal intercondylar area
4	Muscular (extensor) groove	12	Head of fibula	20	Popliteal notch
5	Lateral condyle	13	Facet for proximal articulation with fibula	21	Facet for articulation of sesamoid in tendon M. popliteus
6	Tibial tuberosity	14	Body of fibula	22	Distal articular surface with cochlea of tibia
7	Cranial border (tibial crest)	15	Lateral malleolus		
8	Facies articularis fibularis	16	Facies articulares malleoli		

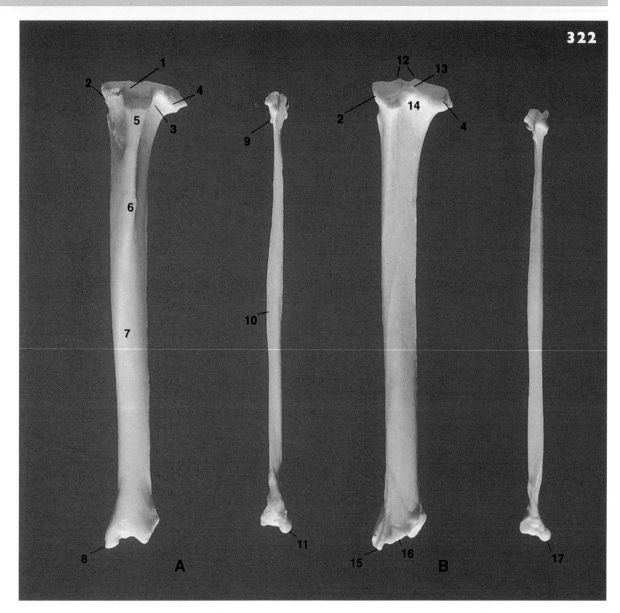

322   Cranial aspect of the left tibia and fibula (A) and caudal aspect of the right tibia and fibula (B) of a cat.

1 Cranial intercondylar area	7 Body of tibia	13 Caudal intercondylar area
2 Medial condyle	8 Medial malleolus	14 Popliteal notch
3 Muscular groove	9 Head } of fibula	15 Medial malleolus of tibia
4 Lateral condyle	10 Body }	16 Distal articular surface
5 Tibial tuberosity	11 Lateral malleolus	17 Lateral malleolus of fibula
6 Cranial border	12 Intercondylar eminence	

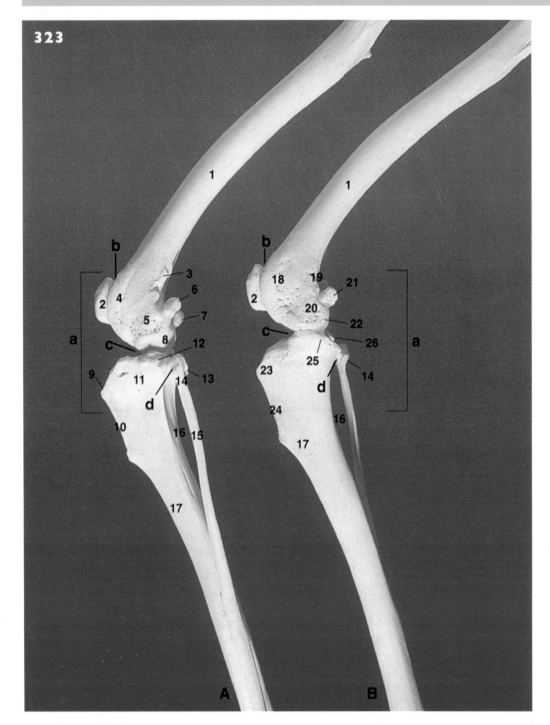

323   Lateral aspect of the left stifle joint and medial aspect of the right stifle joint of a dog.

a Stifle joint	8 Lateral condyle of femur	19 Medial supracondylar
b Femoropatellar joint	9 Tibial tuberosity	tuberosity
c Femorotibial joint	10 Cranial border (tibial crest)	20 Medial epicondyle
d Proximal tibiofibular joint	11 Muscular (extensor) groove	21 Medial fabella
	12 Lateral condyle of tibia	(M. gastrocnemius)
	13 Proximal tibiofibular joint	22 Medial condyle of femur
1 Body of femur	14 Head ⎱ of fibula	23 Tibial crest
2 Patella	15 Body ⎰	24 Cranial border
3 Lateral supracondylar tuberosity	16 Interosseous space	25 Medial condyle of tibia
4 Lateral ridge of trochlea	17 Body of tibia	26 Sesamoid in tendon of
5 Lateral epicondyle	18 Medial ridge of trochlea	M. popliteus
6 Lateral fabella ⎱ (in origin of M.		
7 Medial fabella ⎰ gastrocnemius)		

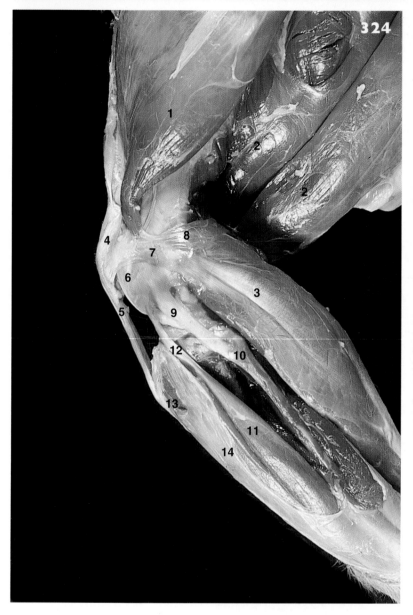

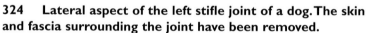

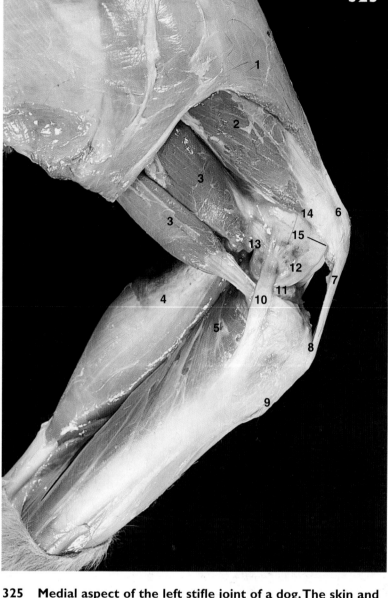

324 **Lateral aspect of the left stifle joint of a dog. The skin and fascia surrounding the joint have been removed.**

325 **Medial aspect of the left stifle joint of a dog. The skin and fascia surrounding the joint have been removed.**

1 M. vastus medialis	8 Site of sesamoid (fabella) in tendon of 3
2 M. semimembranosus	
3 M. gastrocnemius	9 Lateral collateral ligament
4 Patella	10 Fibula
5 Patellar ligament	11 M. extensor digitorum longus
6 Lateral ridge of trochlea	12 Tendon of origin of 11
7 Lateral femoropatellar ligament	13 Tibial tuberosity
	14 M. tibialis cranialis

1 M. sartorius	10 Medial collateral ligament
2 M. vastus medialis	11 Medial meniscus
3 M. semimembranosus	12 Medial condyle of femur
4 M. gastrocnemius	13 Site of sesamoid (fabella) in tendon of 4
5 M. popliteus	
6 Patella	14 Cut edge of femoropatellar ligament
7 Patellar ligament	
8 Tibial tuberosity	15 Medial ridge of trochlea
9 Cranial border (tibial crest)	

326

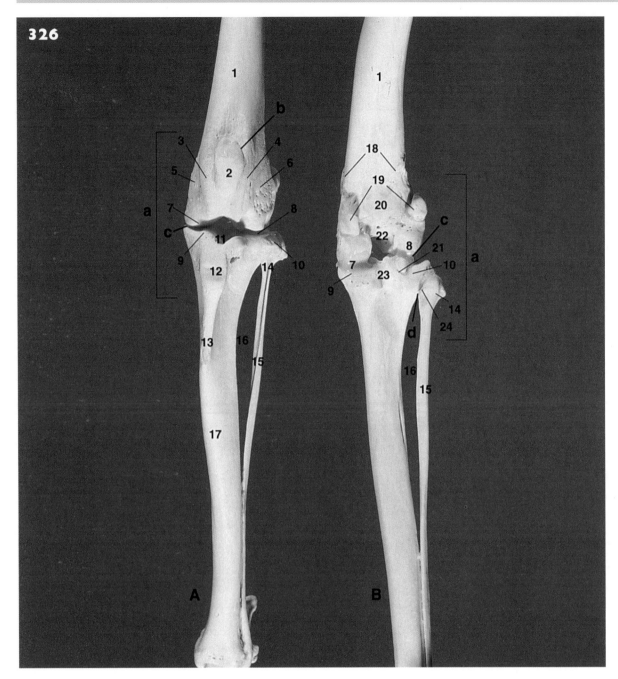

326   Cranial aspect of the left stifle joint (A) and caudal aspect of the right stifle joint (B) of a dog.

a	Stifle joint	
b	Femoropatellar joint	
c	Femorotibial joint	
d	Proximal tibiofibular joint	
1	Body of femur	
2	Patella	
3	Medial ridge } of trochlea	
4	Lateral ridge }	
5	Medial epicondyle } of femur	
6	Lateral epicondyle }	
7	Medial condyle } of femur	
8	Lateral condyle }	
9	Medial condyle } of tibia	
10	Lateral condyle }	
11	Intercondylar area	
12	Tibial tuberosity	
13	Cranial border (tibial crest)	
14	Head } of fibula	
15	Body }	
16	Interosseous space	
17	Body of tibia	
18	Medial and lateral supracondylar tuberosities	
19	Medial and lateral fabellae (in origin of M. gastrocnemius)	
20	Popliteal surface	
21	Sesamoid in tendon of M. popliteus	
22	Intercondylar fossa of femur	
23	Caudal intercondylar area	
24	Proximal tibiofibular joint	

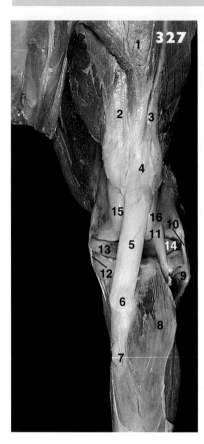

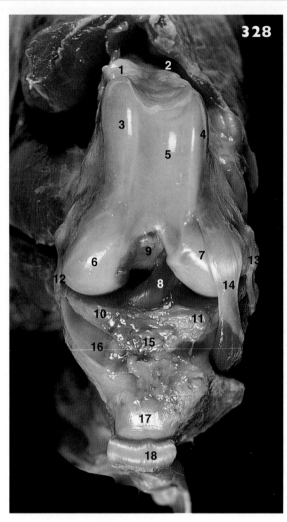

327 Cranial aspect of the left stifle joint of a dog. The skin and fascia surrounding the joint have been removed.

1 M. sartorius
2 M. vastus medialis
3 M. vastus lateralis
4 Patella
5 Patellar ligament
6 Tibial tuberosity
7 Cranial border (tibial crest)
8 M. tibialis cranialis
9 Fibula
10 Lateral collateral ligament
11 Tendon of M. extensor digitorum longus
12 Medial collateral ligament
13 Medial meniscus
14 Lateral meniscus
15 Medial ridge of trochlea
16 Lateral ridge of trochlea

328 Cranial aspect of the left stifle joint of a dog. The patella has been displaced from the trochlea of the femur and retracted distally. The joint has been placed in extreme flexion and the joint capsule opened to reveal the intracapsular structures.

1 Cut joint capsule
2 Sectioned M. quadriceps femoris
3 Medial ridge of trochlea
4 Lateral ridge of trochlea
5 Trochlea
6 Medial condyle of femur
7 Lateral condyle of femur
8 Cranial cruciate ligament
9 Caudal cruciate ligament
10 Medial meniscus
11 Lateral meniscus
12 Medial collateral ligament.
13 Lateral collateral ligament
14 Tendon of M. extensor digitorum longus
15 Infrapatellar fat body
16 Medial condyle of tibia
17 Tibial tuberosity
18 Patellar ligament (reflected)

329 The left stifle joint of a dog after removal of the femur to reveal the articular surface of the proximal extremity of the tibia. The collateral ligaments, the cruciate ligaments and the joint capsule have been transected.

A Caudal
B Cranial

1 Patellar ligament reflected
2 Infrapatellar fat body
3 Transverse ligament
4 Medial meniscus
5 Lateral meniscus
6 Cranial cruciate ligament (cut)
7 Caudal cruciate ligament (cut)
8 Meniscofemoral ligament (cut)
9 Tendon of M. extensor digitorum longus (cut)
10 Lateral collateral ligament (cut)
11 Medial collateral ligament (cut)

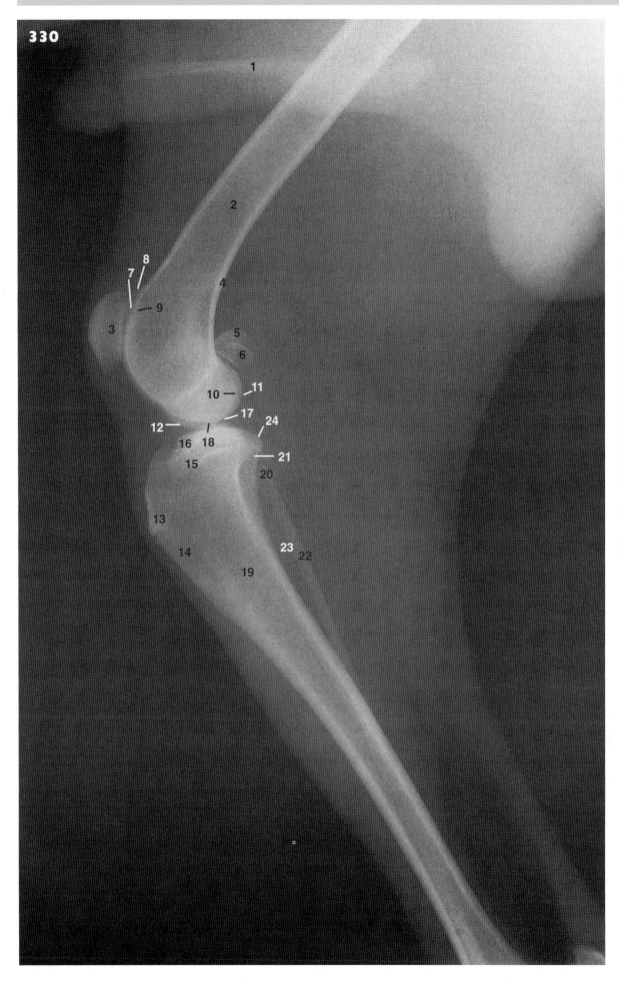

330

330 Mediolateral radiograph of the stifle joint of a dog.

1   Os penis
2   Body of femur
3   Patella
4   Lateral supracondylar tuberosity
5   Lateral fabella ⎫
6   Medial fabella ⎬ (in origin of M. gastrocnemius)
7   Femoropatellar joint
8   Lateral ridge ⎫ of trochlea
9   Medial ridge ⎬
10 Lateral condyle ⎫ of femur
11 Medial condyle ⎬
12 Femorotibial joint
13 Tibial tuberosity
14 Cranial border (tibial crest)
15 Lateral condyle ⎫ of tibia
16 Medial condyle ⎬
17 Lateral intercondylar tubercle
18 Medial intercondylar tubercle
19 Body of tibia
20 Head of fibula
21 Proximal tibiofibular joint
22 Body of fibula
23 Interosseous space
24 Fabella in the tendon of M. popliteus

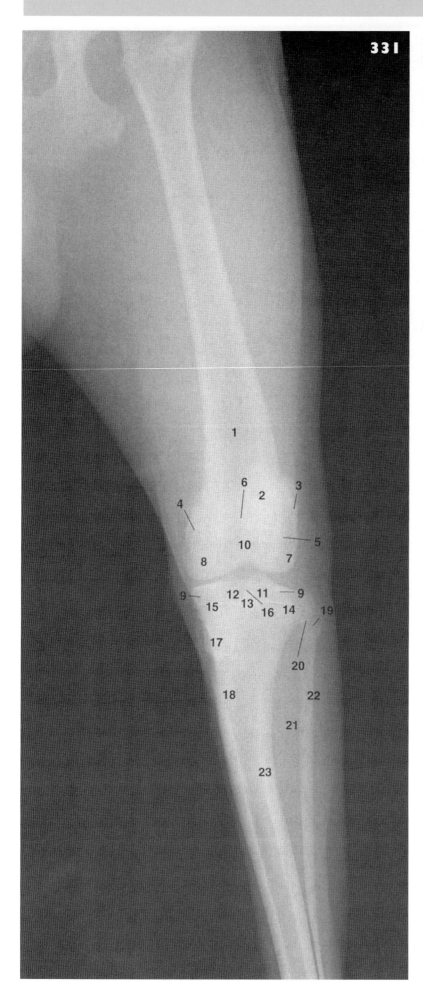

331

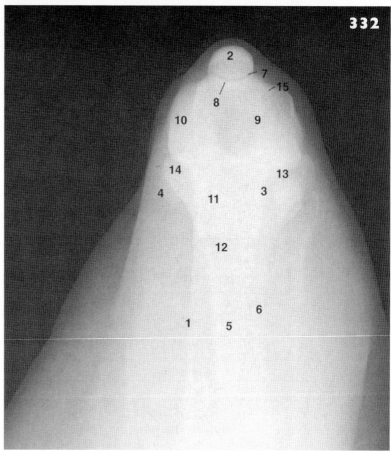

332

331 Craniocaudal radiograph of the stifle joint of a dog.

332 Radiograph of the flexed stifle joint of a dog.

1	Body of femur
2	Patella
3	Lateral fabella (in origin of
4	Medial fabella M. gastrocnemius)
5	Lateral ridge of trochlea
6	Medial ridge
7	Lateral condyle of femur
8	Medial condyle
9	Femorotibial joint space
10	Intercondylar fossa
11	Lateral intercondylar tubercle
12	Medial intercondylar tubercle
13	Intercondylar area
14	Lateral condyle of tibia
15	Medial condyle
16	Fabella in tendon of M. popliteus
17	Tibial tuberosity
18	Base of tibial crest
19	Head of fibula
20	Proximal tibiofibular joint
21	Interosseous space
22	Body of fibula
23	Body of tibia

1	Body of femur
2	Patella
3	Lateral fabella (in origin of
4	Medial fabella M. gastrocnemius)
5	Body of tibia
6	Body of fibula
7	Femoropatellar joint
8	Trochlear groove
9	Lateral condyle of femur
10	Medial condyle
11	Tibial tuberosity
12	Cranial border (tibial crest)
13	Lateral condyle of tibia
14	Medial condyle
15	Extensor fossa

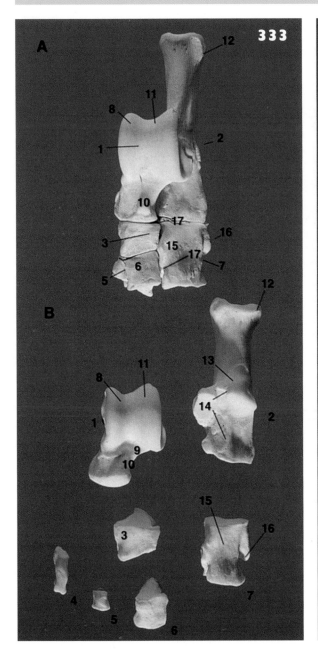

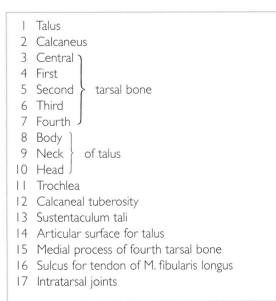

333 Dorsal aspect of the articulated (A) and separated (B) left tarsus of a dog.

1	Talus
2	Calcaneus
3	Central ⎫
4	First ⎪
5	Second ⎬ tarsal bone
6	Third ⎪
7	Fourth ⎭
8	Body ⎫
9	Neck ⎬ of talus
10	Head ⎭
11	Trochlea
12	Calcaneal tuberosity
13	Sustentaculum tali
14	Articular surface for talus
15	Medial process of fourth tarsal bone
16	Sulcus for tendon of M. fibularis longus
17	Intratarsal joints

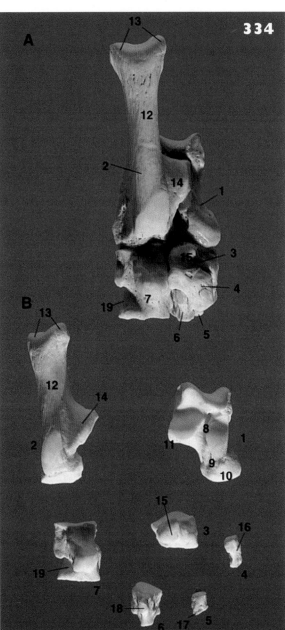

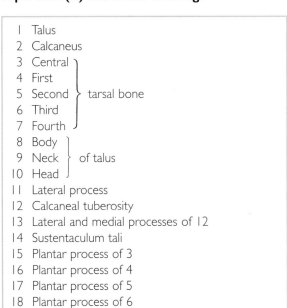

334 Plantar aspect of the articulated (A) and separated (B) left tarsus of a dog.

1	Talus
2	Calcaneus
3	Central ⎫
4	First ⎪
5	Second ⎬ tarsal bone
6	Third ⎪
7	Fourth ⎭
8	Body ⎫
9	Neck ⎬ of talus
10	Head ⎭
11	Lateral process
12	Calcaneal tuberosity
13	Lateral and medial processes of 12
14	Sustentaculum tali
15	Plantar process of 3
16	Plantar process of 4
17	Plantar process of 5
18	Plantar process of 6
19	Sulcus for tendon of M. fibularis longus

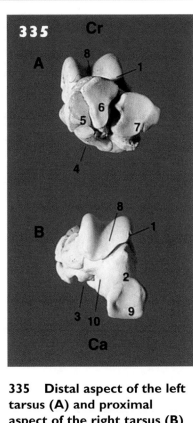

335 Distal aspect of the left tarsus (A) and proximal aspect of the right tarsus (B) of a dog. Cranial (Cr) and caudal (Ca) orientations are indicated.

1	Talus
2	Calcaneus
3	Central ⎫
4	First ⎪
5	Second ⎬ tarsal bone
6	Third ⎪
7	Fourth ⎭
8	Proximal trochlea
9	Calcaneal tuberosity
10	Sustentaculum tali

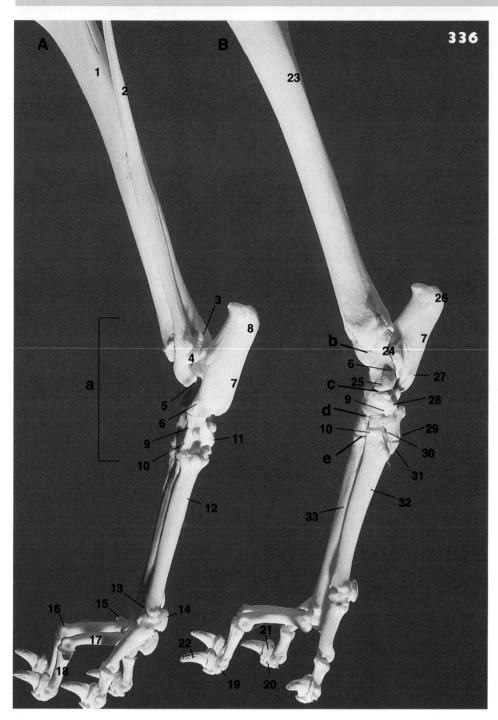

336 **Lateral aspect of the left tarsus and pes (A) and medial aspect of the right tarsus and pes (B) of a dog.**

a	Tarsal joints	9	Central ⎫	20	Distal phalanx
b	Talocrural joint	10	Third ⎬ tarsal bone	21	Ungual crest
c	Proximal intertarsal	11	Fourth ⎭	22	Ungual process
	joint	12	Fifth metatarsal bone	23	Tibia
d	Distal intertarsal joint	13	Metatarsophalangeal	24	Medial malleolus
e	Tarsometatarsal joints		joint	25	Neck of talus
		14	Proximal sesamoids	26	Calcaneal tuberosity
1	Body of tibia		(plantar)	27	Sulcus for flexors
2	Body of fibula	15	Dorsal sesamoids	28	Plantar process of 9
3	Distal tibiofibular joint	16	Proximal	29	First ⎫
4	Lateral malleolus		interphalangeal joint	30	Second ⎬ tarsal bone
5	Trochlea ⎫	17	Proximal phalanx	31	First ⎫
6	Body ⎬ of talus	18	Middle phalanx	32	Second ⎬ metatarsal bone
7	Calcaneus	19	Distal interphalangeal	33	Third ⎭
8	Calcaneal tuberosity		joint		

337 **Mediolateral radiograph of the tarsal joint and pes of a dog.**

1	Body of tibia	17	Medial malleolus
2	Body of fibula	18	Cochlea of tibia
3	Talus	19	Trochlea of talus
4	Calcaneus	20	Calcaneal tuberosity
5	Central ⎫	21	Sustenaculum tali
6	First ⎪	22	Proximal sesamoids
7	Second ⎬ tarsal bone	23	Dorsal sesamoid
8	Third ⎪	24	Metatarsophalangeal
9	Fourth ⎭		joint
10	First metatarsal bone	25	Proximal phalanx
11	Second to fifth	26	Middle phalanx
	metatarsal bones	27	Distal phalanx
12	Talocrural joint	28	Proximal
13	Proximal intertarsal		interphalangeal joint
	joint	29	Distal interphalangeal
14	Distal intertarsal joint		joint
15	Tarsometatarsal joint	30	Ungual crest
16	Lateral malleolus		

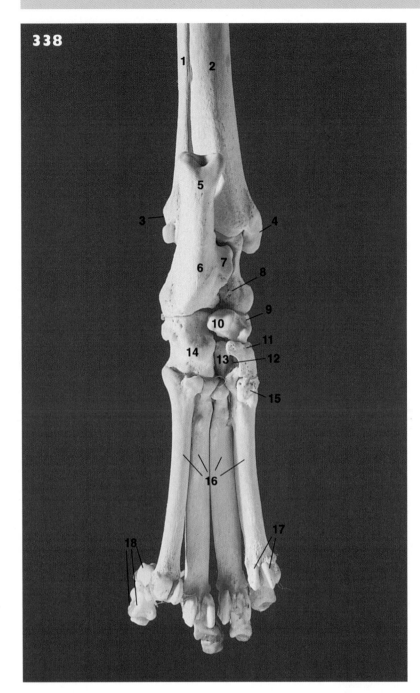

338   Plantar aspect of the tarsal joint and pes of a dog.

1	Fibula	11	First ⎫
2	Tibia	12	Second ⎬ tarsal bone
3	Lateral malleolus	13	Third ⎭
4	Medial malleolus	14	Fourth
5	Calcaneal tuberosity	15	First metatarsal bone
6	Calcaneus	16	Second to fifth metatarsal
7	Sustentaculum tall		bones
8	Talus	17	Proximal sesamoids
9	Central tarsal bone	18	Proximal, middle and distal
10	Plantar process of 9		phalanges

339   Dorsoplantar radiograph of the tarsal joint and pes of a dog.

1	Body of tibia
2	Body of fibula
3	Talus
4	Calcaneus
5	Central ⎫
6	First ⎪
7	Second ⎬ tarsal bone
8	Third ⎪
9	Fourth ⎭
10	First ⎫
11	Second ⎪
12	Third ⎬ metatarsal bone
13	Fourth ⎪
14	Fifth ⎭
15	Talocrural joint
16	Proximal intertarsal joint
17	Distal intertarsal joint
18	Tarsometatarsal joint
19	Lateral malleolus
20	Medial malleolus
21	Dorsal border
22	Lateral groove ⎫ of cochlea
23	Medial groove ⎭ of tibia
24	Lateral ridge ⎫ of trochlea
25	Medial ridge ⎭ of talus
26	Groove
27	Calcaneal tuberosity
28	Sustentaculum tali
29	Proximal sesamoids
30	Metatarsophalangeal joint
31	Outline of metatarsal pad
32	Proximal phalanx
33	Proximal interphalangeal joint
34	Middle phalanx
35	Distal interphalangeal joint
36	Distal phalanx
37	Ungual crest
38	Ungual process

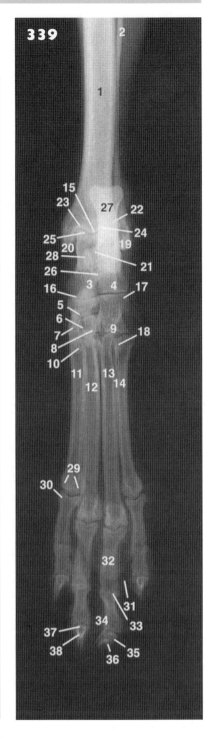

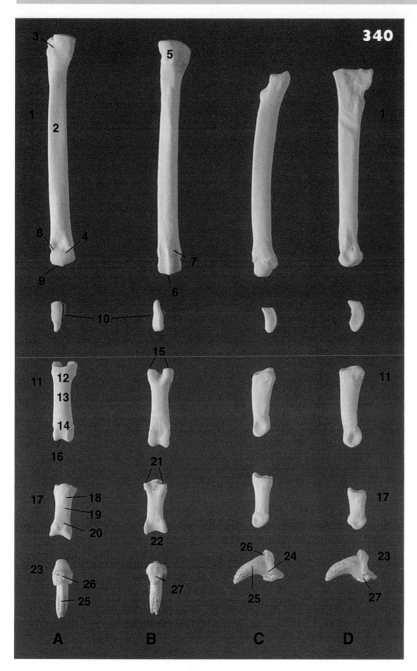

340   Dorsal (A), plantar (B), abaxial (C) and axial (D) aspects of a typical digit in the pes of a dog.

1	Metatarsal bone	
2	Body	}
3	Base	} of 1
4	Head	}
5	Plantar tubercles	
6	Sagittal crest	
7	Proximal sesamoid impression	
8	Dorsal sesamoid fossa	
9	Trochlea of 1	
10	Proximal sesamoid	
11	Proximal phalanx	
12	Base	}
13	Body	}
14	Head	} of 11
15	Plantar tubercles	}
16	Trochlea	}
17	Middle phalanx	
18	Base	}
19	Body	}
20	Head	} of 17
21	Plantar tubercles	}
22	Trochlea	}
23	Distal phalanx	
24	Body of 23	
25	Ungual process	
26	Ungual crest	
27	Insertion of M. flexor digitorum profundus	

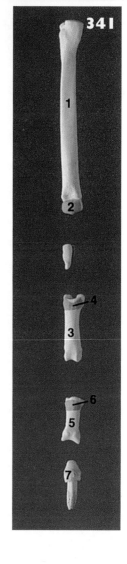

341   Dorsal aspect of a typical digit in the pes of a dog, showing the centres of ossification.

1 Body of metatarsal bone
2 Distal
3 Body of proximal phalanx
4 Proximal
5 Body of middle phalanx
6 Proximal
7 Body of distal phalanx

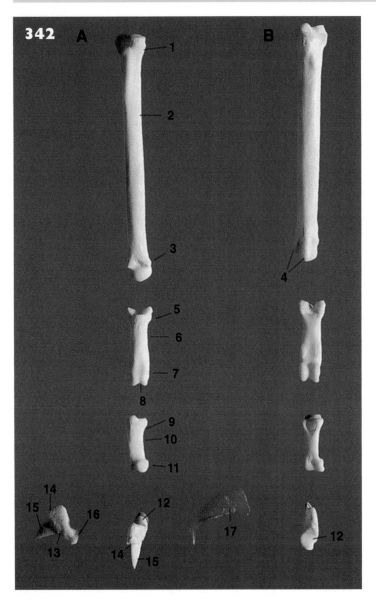

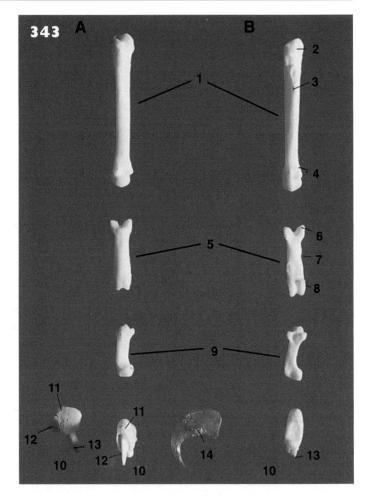

342   Dorsal (A) and plantar (B) aspects of a typical digit in the pes of a cat. The lateral aspects of the distal phalanx and the claw are also displayed.

1	Base ⎫	12	Base ⎫ of distal phalanx
2	Body ⎬ of metatarsal bone	13	Body ⎭
3	Head ⎭	14	Ungual crest
4	Sesamoid impression	15	Ungual process
5	Base ⎫	16	Tubercle for insertion of M.
6	Body ⎬ of proximal phalanx		flexor digitorum profundus
7	Head ⎭	17	Claw (unguis)
8	Trochlea		
9	Base ⎫		
10	Body ⎬ of middle phalanx		
11	Head ⎭		

343   Dorsal (A) and palmar (B) aspects of a typical digit in the manus of a cat. The lateral aspects of the distal phalanx and the claw are also displayed.

1	Metacarpal bone	9	Middle phalanx
2	Base ⎫	10	Distal phalanx
3	Body ⎬ of metacarpal bone	11	Ungual crest
4	Head ⎭	12	Ungual process
5	Proximal phalanx	13	Tubercle for insertion of
6	Base ⎫		M. flexor digitorum profundus
7	Body ⎬ of first phalanx	14	Claw (unguis)
8	Head ⎭		

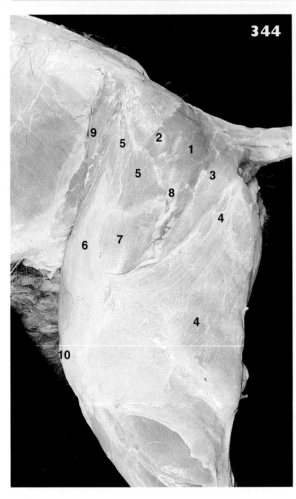

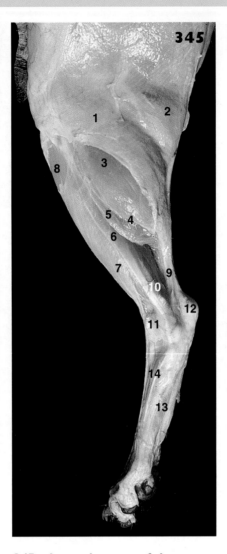

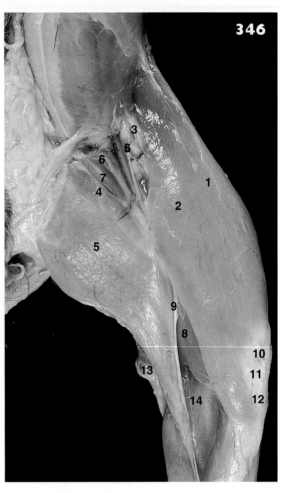

344   Lateral aspect of the pelvic and thigh regions of the left pelvic limb of a cat.

1 M. gluteus superficialis
2 M. gluteus medius
3 M. caudofemoralis
4 M. biceps femoris
5 M. tensor fasciae latae
6 Fascia lata
7 M. vastus lateralis
8 Greater trochanter
9 M. sartorius
10 Patella

345   Lateral aspect of the crus and pes of the left pelvic limb of a cat.

1 Tendon of M. biceps femoris
2 M. semitendinosus
3 M. gastrocnemius
4 M. flexor digitorum superficialis
5 M. soleus
6 M. peroneus longus
7 M. extensor digitorum longus
8 M. tibialis cranialis
9 Tendo calcaneus communis (Achilles)
10 M. peroneus brevis
11 Distal extensor retinaculum
12 Calcaneal tuberosity
13 Mm. interossei
14 M. extensor digitorum brevis

346   Medial aspect of the pelvic and thigh regions of the left pelvic limb of a cat.

1 Cranial part of M. sartorius
2 Caudal part of M. sartorius
3 Tendon of M. rectus femoris
4 Mm. adductores
5 M. gracilis
6 Femoral triangle (with femoral artery, vein and saphenous nerve)
7 M. pectineus
8 M. semimembranosus
9 Medial saphenous vein
10 Patella
11 Patellar ligament
12 Tibial tuberosity
13 Popliteal lymph node
14 M. gastrocnemius

347

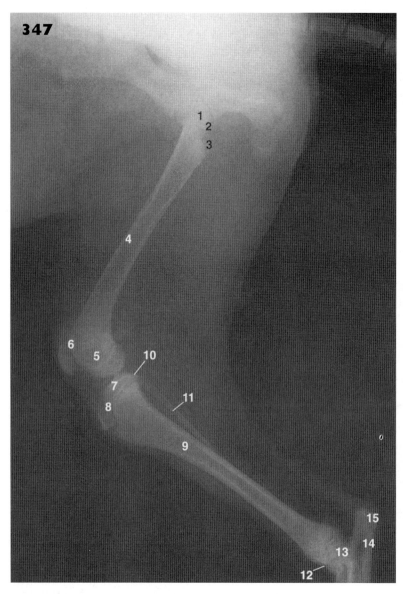

347   Mediolateral radiograph of the thigh region, stifle and tarsal joint of a puppy, showing the centres of ossification.

1	Head of femur	9	Body of tibia
2	Greater trochanter	10	Proximal epiphysis ⎫
3	Lesser trochanter	11	Body ⎬ of fibula
4	Body ⎫ of femur	12	Distal epiphysis ⎭
5	Distal epiphysis ⎭	13	Distal epiphysis of tibia
6	Patella	14	Body of calcaneus
7	Proximal tibial epiphysis	15	Calcaneal tuberosity
8	Cranial border (tibial crest)		

Clinical Note
8   The tibial crest has its own centre of ossification separated from the body by a cartilaginous growth plate. As the tendon of insertion of the M. quadriceps inserts here by means of the straight patellar ligament, this centre can become distracted from the body – requiring surgical correction.

348

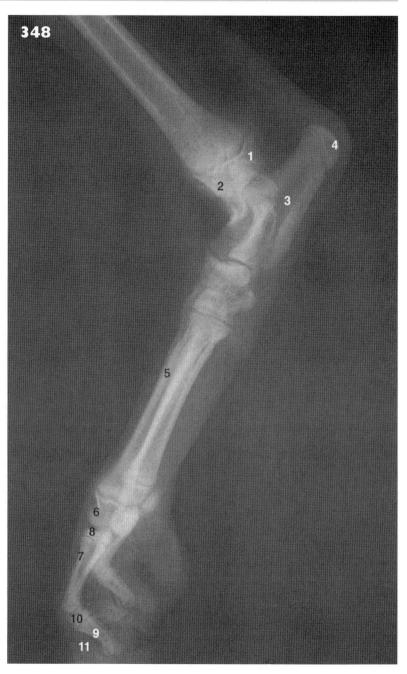

348   Mediolateral radiograph of the tarsal joint and pes of a puppy, showing the centres of ossification.

1	Distal epiphysis of tibia	7	Body ⎫ of proximal
2	Distal epiphysis of fibula	8	Proximal ⎬ phalanx
3	Body of calcaneus		epiphysis ⎭
4	Calcaneal tuberosity	9	Body ⎫ of middle
5	Body ⎫ of	10	Proximal epiphysis ⎭ phalanx
6	Distal epiphysis ⎭ metatarsus	11	Body of distal phalanx

Clinical Note
4   The calcaneal tuberosity has its own centre of ossification separated from the body of the calcaneus by a growth plate. As the common calcanean tendon inserts here, this centre can become distracted from the body – requiring surgical correction.

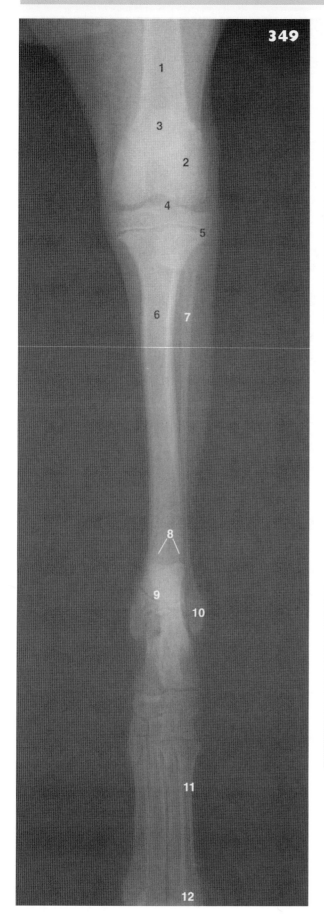

349

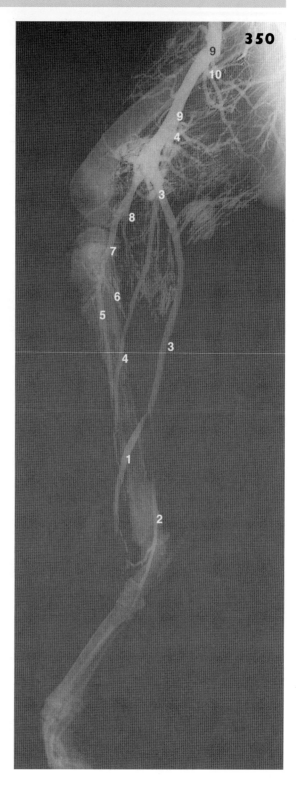

350

349 Craniocaudal dorsoplantar radiograph of the stifle and tarsal joint of a puppy, showing the centres of ossification.

1	Body } of femur
2	Distal epiphysis
3	Patella
4	Proximal epiphysis of tibia
5	Proximal epiphysis of fibula
6	Body of tibia
7	Body of fibula
8	Calcaneal tuberosity
9	Distal epiphysis of tibia
10	Distal epiphysis of fibula
11	Body of metatarsus
12	Distal epiphysis

350 Mediolateral radiograph of a venogram of the pelvic limb of a dog.

1	Cranial branch } of lateral
2	Caudal branch } saphenous vein
3	Lateral saphenous vein
4	Medial saphenous vein
5	Cranial tibial vein
6	Caudal tibial vein
7	Popliteal vein
8	Distal caudal femoral vein
9	Femoral vein
10	Deep femoral vein

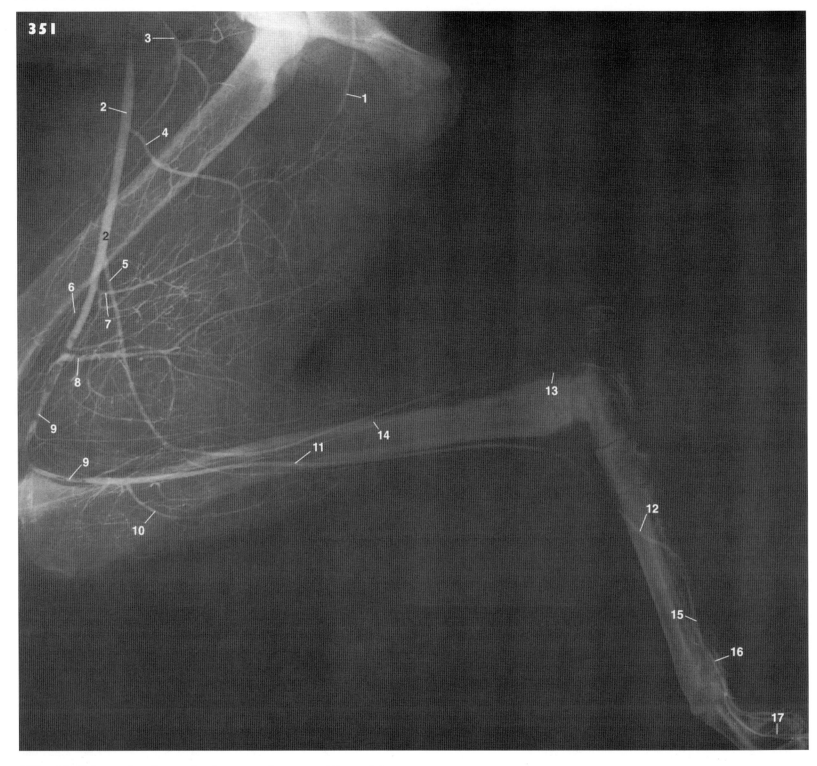

351   Mediolateral radiograph of an arteriogram of the pelvic limb of a dog.

1	Caudal gluteal artery from internal iliac artery	8	Distal caudal femoral artery
		9	Popliteal artery
2	Femoral artery from external iliac artery	10	Caudal tibial artery
		11	Cranial tibial artery
3	Lateral circumflex femoral artery	12	Perforating metatarsal artery
		13	Caudal branch
4	Proximal caudal femoral artery	14	Cranial branch } of 5
5	Saphenous artery	15	Plantar metatarsal arteries
6	Descending genicular artery	16	Plantar common digital arteries
7	Middle caudal femoral artery	17	Plantar proper digital arteries

INDEX

Numbers refer to Figures. References are to adult dogs, unless otherwise stated.